Super Foods for a
Super Healthy You

Unleash the secret healing power
of Nature's ultimate foods

By Rachael Linkie

... Including 57 delicious recipes
for every occasion

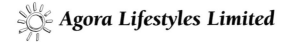

Agora Lifestyles Limited

If you have any queries, please contact Customer Services at: Agora Lifestyles Ltd, 7th Floor, Sea Containers House, 20 Upper Ground, London SE1 9JD. You may also call 020 7633 3630 or send a fax to 020 7633 3740.

ISBN No: 978-0-9560100-0-1

CONTENTS

Introduction: The medicine chest in your food – How to
look and feel better than you have done in years . . . . .Page 1

Chapter 1: Fruit – How colour is integral to unlocking
its diverse range of health benefits . . . . .Page 7

Açaí: Nature's perfect food – The amazing health benefits
of the fruit from the Amazon's 'tree of life' . . . . .Page 10

Refreshing açaí and mango smoothie . . . . .Page 13

An apple a day really can help keep your doctor away . . . . .Page 14

Pork chops with apple sauce . . . . .Page 15

How diet remains one of the number 1 antidotes to
the ageing process . . . . .Page 16

Research findings uncover cancer-fighting properties
linked to avocados . . . . .Page 18

Spicy avocado dip to wake up your taste buds . . . . .Page 19

The bountiful benefits of bananas . . . . .Page 20

Banana and raisin bread . . . . .Page 21

Blueberries can protect your brain cells, beat cystitis and
stop cancer in its tracks . . . . .Page 22

Mouthwatering blueberry muffins . . . . .Page 26

Cherries provide a vital defence against Type 2 diabetes
and cardiovascular disease . . . . .Page 27

Cherry sorbet – for the occasional tasty treat . . . . .Page 30

Cranberries can help fight antibiotic-resistant
urinary tract infections . . . . .Page 31

Festive cranberry sauce – the perfect accompaniment to turkey . .Page 35

How the health benefits of oranges extend beyond vitamin C . . . .Page 35

Orange and lemon roasted chicken . . . . .Page 36

Eat more pineapple to maintain good joint health . . . . .Page 37

Simple-to-prepare pineapple salsa . . . . .Page 38

The remarkable anti-cancer and anti-inflammatory
properties linked to pomegranates . . . . .Page 39

The dark purple smoothie loaded with antioxidants . . . . .Page 45

Raspberries offer a simple way to protect against cancer . . . . . . .Page 46

Berry bliss smoothie . . . . .Page 47

Tomatoes – Why tomato sauce could protect men
from prostate cancer . . . . .Page 48

Ratatouille – A traditional, tasty way to benefit from tomatoes . . .Page 49

Discover how an Asian plum – relied upon by legendary
samurai warriors to boost their stamina and energy levels –
could benefit your health . . . . .Page 50

Delicious vegetarian sushi rolls . . . . .Page 53

Chapter 2: Vegetables – In a league of their own when it
comes to providing essential nutrients .Page 55

Ashitaba – News about this 'super food' from Japan is quickly
spreading... make sure you don't miss out on its many benefits . . .Page 58

Eat your greens and your blood pressure will drop . . . . .Page 62

How beetroot is making a comeback . . . . .Page 62

Beetroot soup – A delicious way to cleanse your system . . . . . . .Page 65

Broccoli provides you with an important defence
against stomach ulcers and cancer . . . . .Page 66

Spicy chicken and broccoli dish . . . . .Page 67

The top 20 antioxidant vegetables . . . . .Page 68

Garlic – How to make sure you're taking full advantage
of its heart-friendly properties . . . . .Page 69

Steamed garlic and lemon grass sea bass . . . . .Page 72

Mushrooms possess a wide range of therapeutic actions . . . . . . .Page 72

Mixed oriental mushroom risotto . . . . .Page 74

Onions can protect your bones and help prevent osteoporosis . . .Page 75

Go continental with a delicious French onion tart . . . . .Page 77

Don't overlook the merits of the humble potato... especially
the sweet variety . . . . .Page 78

Vegetarian shepherd's pie with sweet potato . . . . .Page 80

Good news for Type 1 diabetics: adding pumpkin to your
diet could help regulate your blood sugar levels . . . . .Page 81

Hearty pumpkin, pepper and coriander soup . . . . .Page 83

Spinach is packed with important, disease-fighting nutrients . . . .Page 84

Spinach, avocado and beetroot salad . . . . .Page 85

Researchers reveal how watercress plays a vital role in
the prevention of cancer . . . . .Page 86

Watercress and goat's cheese salad . . . . .Page 88

Chapter 3: Grains – How to make sure you're eating
the right kind . . . . .Page 91

Fibre could help postmenopausal women lower their
cholesterol... and lose inches from their hips and waist . . . . .Page 92

The difference between soluble and insoluble fibre . . . . .Page 96

Savoury brown rice nutty salad . . . . .Page 98

Quinoa and tofu loaf. . . . . .Page 98

Spiced prawn, avocado and bulgar wheat salad with
salmon pancake rolls . . . . .Page 99

Kick-start your day with a refreshing fruit and oat smoothie . . . .Page 100

Chapter 4: Seeds, beans and pulses – A good source of
protein, fibre, vitamins and minerals . . . . .Page 103

Soy – Boosting your intake could reduce your risk of cancer . . .Page 104

How to benefit from hemp seed's perfect balance of
omega-3 and omega-6 fatty acids . . . . .Page 105

Salba seeds – This Aztec staple can help overcome
everything from constipation to high blood sugar levels . . . . . . .Page 106

Fill up on these nutritious seeds and pulses too . . . . .Page 110

Comforting lentil and tomato soup . . . . .Page 111

Hearty split pea soup . . . . .Page 111

Tuna and butter bean salad . . . . .Page 112

Mushroom and miso soup . . . . .Page 113

Chickpea casserole with spinach . . . . .Page 114

Chapter 5: Herbs and spices add flavour and health-promoting
properties to your food . . . . .Page 117

Basil: A simple way to maintain the health of your heart . . . . . .Page 117

Cod in tomato and basil sauce . . . . .Page 119

Cinnamon: Discover how an ordinary kitchen spice led
to the development of an extraordinary diabetes remedy . . . . . . .Page 120

Quick and delicious banana and cinnamon smoothie . . . . .Page 123

Fennel: Far more than a simple recipe ingredient...
it helps fight everything from infections to obesity . . . . .Page 123

Fresh fennel and walnut salad . . . . .Page 126

Ginger: The herb with a diverse range of therapeutic actions . . .Page 127

Prawn and veggie ginger stir-fry . . . . .Page 128

Instant energy ginger juice . . . . .Page 129

Oregano: The herb that's generating a great deal of
excitement in the scientific community for its ability
to treat everything from urinary to fungal infections . . . . .Page 130

Black olives with oregano . . . . .Page 133

Rosemary: The well-known herb with hidden benefits...
including an ability to prevent cancer . . . . .Page 133

Rosemary chicken with a kick . . . . .Page 137

Turmeric: Helps reduce the number and severity of IBS
attacks... meaning less abdominal pain and bloating . . . . .Page 138

Spicy pumpkin curry with turmeric . . . . .Page 141

Chapter 6: Nuts: The snack that can benefit your health in numerous ways... from preventing heart disease to boosting immunity . . . .Page 143

Eating walnuts can protect your arteries... even following
a high-fat meal . . . . .Page 144

Broccoli and walnut salad with apple vinaigrette sauce . . . . . . .Page 146

Chunky nut and vegetable roast . . . . .Page 147

Chapter 7: Fats: Separating the good from the bad . . . . .Page 149

Including more olive oil in your diet could help lower
your risk of cancer . . . . .Page 150

Virgin coconut oil: The unique saturated fat that
actually promotes weight loss . . . . .Page 153

Sautéed sea bass with virgin coconut oil and garlic . . . . .Page 156

Roasted vegetables in extra virgin olive oil with couscous . . . . . .Page 157

Chapter 8: Fish has proven protective benefits for
many of your body's most important organs . . . . .Page 159

This spicy mackerel dish provides a tasty way to top
up your levels of omega-3 . . . . .Page 162

Salmon with a tangy, mango salsa twist . . . . .Page 164

Grilled oysters in lemon butter . . . . .Page 165

Monkfish and veggie mix . . . . .Page 166

Salad niçoise . . . . .Page 167

Chapter 9: Meat helps provide your body with fuel . . . . .Page 169

Warming turkey chilli . . . . .Page 170

Chicken caesar salad . . . . .Page 171

Pork and spinach sesame seed stir-fry . . . . .Page 172

Chapter 10: Dairy products: uncovering common
myths, particularly when it comes to milk . . . . .Page 173

Cut your blood pressure in half by eating low-fat dairy . . . . . . .Page 174

Men – Lower your risk of the 3rd most common cancer
by eating more calcium and dairy . . . . .Page 176

Grilled salmon fillets with a herb yoghurt sauce . . . . .Page 178

Pepper, lentil and goat's cheese surprise . . . . .Page 179

Chapter 11: Eggs – Don't let anyone try and tell
you they're bad for your heart! . . . . .Page 181

Asparagus and sautéed mushroom filled omelette . . . . .Page 182

Eggs Florentine and haddock . . . . .Page 183

Chapter 12: Honey – Discover the incredible healing
honey that is showing potential against deadly hospital
super bugs like MRSA . . . . .Page 185

Honey more effective than many cough medicines . . . . .Page 187

Roasted veg with manuka honey and feta cheese . . . . .Page 189

Chapter 13: Sugar – How too much can increase your
risk of a stroke, heart attack and diabetes . . . . .Page 191

Flavonoids found in dark chocolate help lower
high blood pressure . . . . .Page 192

Indulgent chocolate and walnut mousse . . . . .Page 194

Chapter 14: Why not all super foods are healthy
for everyone . . . . .Page 197

Chapter 15: Is organic food really better? . . . . .Page 201

Chapter 16: The way you cook your food can be
just as important as the foods you opt for . . . . .Page 205

Make sure your cooking utensils and tap water
aren't damaging your brain . . . . .Page 205

Microwaves: They're convenient, they're fast,
but are they really safe? . . . . .Page 207

Chapter 17: Drink your way to good health . . . . .Page 211

Water can affect the amount of nutrients your body's
getting from the food you eat . . . . .Page 211

Coffee: Is your morning cup making you feel rundown
and ill-tempered? . . . . .Page 217

Coffee berries and pomegranates – The unusual duo that
together provide superior antioxidant action . . . . .Page 217

Tea: Numerous benefits linked to your morning cup of tea . . . .Page 222

The compound that a leading Harvard medical professor
believes 'could potentially get rid of 4 out of the 5 most
common diseases in the Western world' . . . . .Page 232

Alcohol can be a major obstacle in the battle to lose weight . . . .Page 234

A new study shows that substances found in beer, wine
and tea could prevent the spread of breast cancer . . . . .Page 236

A final word of advice . . . . .Page 239

Further reading . . . . .Page 240

Helpful organisations . . . . .Page 242

Your helpful recipe guide at a glance . . . . .Page 243

Tasty meals and drinks you can rustle up in 15 minutes or less . .Page 243

Winter warmers – The perfect comfort foods . . . . .Page 244

When the temperature rises try these delicious
summertime dishes . . . . .Page 245

Vegetarian super food options . . . . .Page 246

Meals for special occasions and entertaining . . . . .Page 247

Index . . . . .Page 249

INTRODUCTION:

The medicine chest in your food – How to look and feel better than you have done in years

You've probably read or heard the phrase "Let food be thy medicine". Uttered by Hippocrates, 'the Father of Medicine', more than 2,000 years ago, today his famous words now hold more truth and credibility than ever before. This follows extensive scientific research that is continually uncovering incredible health-related benefits linked to a wide range of foods from all over the globe.

Foods that fall into the 'super food' category are those that contain high amounts of beneficial substances like vitamins, minerals and enzymes that boost your immune system, increase your energy levels, help your body get rid of harmful toxins, and protect you from illness.

For example, did you know that cinnamon – the ingredient used to flavour a variety of dishes and that you probably have sitting on your kitchen spice rack – can help regulate your blood sugar levels and ward off diabetes? Or that simply by eating a handful of nuts a few times a week you could reduce your risk of getting a heart attack by at least 15 per cent and perhaps by as much as 51 per cent?

Oily fish – the heart protective properties of which have been well-documented – is another star player that rates highly on the super food list. But what you might not be aware of is research that shows how eating oily fish as little as once a week could lower your risk of Alzheimer's by a staggering 60 per cent.

Eating more foods like these, which deliver a nutrition-packed punch with every serving, has never been so important. This is especially true given that many chronic diseases, such as diabetes, heart disease, osteoarthritis and cancer are on the increase in developed countries. What makes this situation so tragic is that in many cases these diseases are entirely preventable... simply by eating the right kind of foods and taking regular exercise.

Is your diet slowly killing you?

Take cancer, for example. The World Health Organization (WHO) has revealed that 85 per cent of adult cancers are entirely avoidable and, of these, around half are related to nutritional deficiencies in the Western diet.

By contrast, an impressive body of research has revealed that those people who eat the recommended serving of five fruits and vegetables a day (as a minimum) are half as likely to develop cancer as those who eat the least amount of these foods.

What you don't eat is just as important as what you do eat. The latest research findings have revealed that consuming too many processed meats can increase the risk of bowel and pancreatic cancer. In fact, eating just one sausage a day increases your risk of bowel cancer by up to 20 per cent.

Diabetes is another case in point. A sedentary lifestyle, combined with a diet high in refined carbohydrates and sugary foods is largely to blame for the rapid increase in Type 2 diabetes. In fact, Type 2 diabetes is commonly referred to as 'maturity-onset diabetes', because most people who get it are over 40 and overweight.

Many people are leaving themselves incredibly vulnerable to obesity and a lifetime of ill-health as a result of their heavy reliance on junk food and chemically treated, processed foods. As well as having little (if any) nutritional value they're typically laden with too much fat, refined sugar and salt, not to mention all the artificial colourings, flavourings and preservatives.

This leaves your poor body overwhelmed with the task of getting rid of all these harmful toxins, which places a huge burden on important organs like your liver and kidneys. As a result your body has less time to get on with its usual important tasks of cleansing, healing and renewal.

If you followed every bit of dietary advice you read about, you'd end up eating nothing!

The need for sound dietary advice has never been greater. Especially given that there is so much confusing and conflicting dietary information out there. One minute we're told to steer clear of a certain food as it can cause X, Y and Z conditions and the next to eat more of it.

Take alcohol for instance. First it's bad for us, then we're being told we should be drinking a couple of glasses a day to prevent heart disease. Don't let's even get started on the whole fat debate! Do you risk spreading your toast with the cancer-causing trans fats in margarine or the artery-clogging saturated fats in butter?

No wonder we're all confused! Trying to sort out the myths from the facts is an arduous task for most nutritionists nowadays... let alone the rest of us!

It doesn't help matters that the media cashes in on our fear and confusion by running with alarmist, scare-mongering and often misleading headlines – like 'a high fat diet causes cancer'... without giving you even half the facts.

Life-altering super foods are available in your local supermarket right now

That's where *Super Foods for a Super Healthy You* can help. You'll discover the very best foods you should be eating more of to help maintain good health, promote weight loss, increase your energy levels, prevent and treat many age-related diseases and help you live longer.

Take celery, for example, which is an excellent source of vitamin C that helps support your immune system. In addition, the chemical that gives celery its distinctive smell – 3-n-butyl phthalide – relaxes the smooth muscle lining of blood vessels, thereby widening the vessels and lowering blood pressure. It also reduces stress hormones, which in turn helps lower high blood pressure. Celery is a diuretic and can therefore help rid your body of excess fluid that reduces the inflammation associated with conditions like arthritis.

Obviously one of the best ways to achieve peak health is to take regular exercise and follow a varied and balanced diet that includes plenty of fresh, wholefoods – choosing organic and seasonal foods whenever possible. It should be rich in whole grains, nuts, seeds, fruits and vegetables which are high in antioxidants – natural chemicals that bolster your immune system and help fight harmful 'cancer-causing' free radicals.

However, despite having this advice drummed into us and despite our best intentions, all too often we get stuck in a rut where our diet is concerned and eat the same types of foods week in, week out, without ever introducing anything new to our weekly shopping list.

However, by loading your supermarket basket with the foods

outlined in the following pages – some of Mother Nature's finest offerings – you'll be doing your health, not to mention your taste buds, a massive favour. It really is possible to eat healthily without giving up treats, starving yourself or spending hours in the kitchen. In fact, studies show that banning foods or going hungry is a bad idea. Not only will you miss out on vital nutrients – you'll feel deprived and end up craving fatty, sugary foods.

The best thing is, you'll also reap the benefits in numerous other ways... including increased energy levels and visible improvements to your skin, hair and nails. Just wait for those compliments to start rolling in left, right and centre!

How to take advantage of the disease-fighting nutrients in nature's miracle foods

Each section of *Super Foods for a Super Healthy You* tells you which foods, within each particular food group, are the most nutrient-rich and have proven benefits for combating particular health problems, to help you make the best dietary choices possible for overall good health. All of the information provided is backed up by the latest scientific research findings and full references are given.

As you'll see, some foods have been found to be particularly beneficial for boosting your immune system while others can help prevent chronic diseases like osteoporosis, heart disease and cancer.

Better still, you're not left with a long list of foods you should be eating more of without knowing how to incorporate them into your daily diet. You'll receive important cooking and handling tips to ensure you're getting the maximum amount of nutrients from the super foods listed.

In addition you'll discover delicious and simple-to-follow recipes that incorporate these beneficial foods, which the whole family can enjoy. There's a helpful reference guide at the back of *Super Foods for a Super Healthy You*, which groups the recipes listed on the following pages into specific categories.

For example, you'll find quick-to-prepare recipes for when you're in a rush, those that are suitable for vegetarians, recipes to suit the different seasons and those that are perfect for entertaining guests such as indulgent chocolate and walnut mousse. However, while some recipes like the latter do contain sugar (which certainly doesn't rank as a super food!) these are intended to be had as occasional treats only. Better still, you can substitute the sugar with healthier alternatives such as honey, apple juice, or dried fruit in desserts and cakes.

You can also have fun inventing new recipes from the food choices given... experiment and be creative! It can also save you time and money to bulk cook and then freeze extra portions of stews, casseroles, soups and sauces to eat later in the week.

By now you're probably itching to know which 'super foods' will protect your body from illness, detox your system and have it running like a Formula One racing car...

So let's begin with fruits and vegetables, which you probably won't be too surprised to learn offer some of the best dietary choices you can make for optimum health – from the obvious to the less well-known super foods from across the globe.

CHAPTER 1

Fruit – how colour is integral to unlocking its diverse range of health benefits

Fruits are abundant in numerous important vitamins, minerals and antioxidants that are necessary to keep your body healthy. Ensuring you eat a wide variety really is the key to making sure you derive maximum health benefits.

This includes making sure you opt for a selection of different coloured fruits, which provide a broad spectrum of essential nutrients. This advice applies to vegetables too, as you'll see below.

For example, fruit and veg with a blue/purple-black colour, such as plums, blueberries, blackberries, raisins, prunes and aubergines contain health-promoting phytochemicals (natural plant compounds) such as anthocyanins and phenolics, which have disease-fighting and anti-ageing benefits.

And those that are yellow/orange in colour – like peaches, apricots, nectarines, pineapples, mangos, oranges, carrots, butternut squash, sweet potatoes and peppers – contain high amounts of cancer-fighting antioxidants including vitamin C, carotenoids and bioflavonoids. Foods high in these nutrients help bolster your body's defences and, according to the World Cancer Research Fund and the American Institute for Cancer Research, they help reduce the risk of various gut and lung cancers.

Green fruit and veggies such as kiwi fruits, kale, spinach, watercress and peas give you plenty of immune-boosting vitamin C, necessary for great skin, and folate – a B vitamin that protects against birth defects. Plus researchers from the International Medical Center of Japan and the National Institute of Health and Nutrition recently discovered that folate may help ease symptoms of depression in men. After assessing the results of a survey conducted on over 500 subjects, they discovered that men with the highest intake of folate were half as likely to suffer from depression as men with the lowest intake (*"Dietary intake of folate, other B vitamins, and omega-3 polyunsaturated fatty acids in relation to depressive symptoms in Japanese adults," Nutrition 2007; published online ahead of print 03/12/07*).

This study is just one in a growing number highlighting similar connections between folate and mood. For example, a recent review of 11 different studies involving over 15,000 patients conducted by researchers at the University of New York and Hull York Medical Center found a significant link between low folate levels and depression (*"Folate may reduce depression symptoms for men, says study," NutraIngredients (www.nutraingredients.com), 07/12/07*).

Kale, spinach and peas are rich sources of lutein – a pigment in the eye that filters out damaging UV rays. A study conducted at Massachusetts Eye and Ear Infirmary found a high intake of spinach or collard greens (similar to kale) was associated with a substantially reduced risk of age-related blindness. Plus green vegetables such as cabbage, broccoli, kale, Brussels sprouts and watercress contain glucosinolates, which appear to protect against cancer by encouraging the self-destruction of pre-cancerous cells.

For protecting against heart disease, cancer and urinary infections make sure you include plenty of red foods, such as strawberries, cranberries, pink grapefruit, watermelon, pomegranates, red apples, tomatoes and red onions. Red foods are among the richest sources of antioxidants called flavonoids, which may protect against heart disease. And, as you'll learn on page 17, tomatoes and watermelon are important providers of lycopene – a pigment in plants thought to reduce the risk of prostate cancer, according to a report by the World Cancer Research Fund. Turn to page 31 to discover why urinary tract infections are no match against cranberries.

To increase your intake of white produce, which are good for lowering cholesterol, detoxing the body, preventing cancer, and keeping blood pressure healthy, eat more bananas, onions, garlic, shallots, leeks, cucumber, celery, fennel and mushrooms. Vegetables in the onion group contain sulphur compounds, which increase the activity of enzymes that remove toxic substances from the body. Sulphur compounds may also help to lower cholesterol and keep your arteries flexible, thereby lowering your risk of heart disease. White fruits and vegetables are also good sources of potassium, which regulates blood pressure.

How all good things come to those who wait!

While just about every piece of health advice you read recommends lots of fresh fruits and vegetables, if you really want to get the most nutritional value out of them, you might want to adjust your definition of 'fresh'.

According to a study published in the *Journal of Agricultural and Food Chemistry*, some fruits and vegetables actually get better for you after they've been stored for a while. Not long enough for them to spoil, of course. The researchers found that when they stored produce items either at room temperature or in the refrigerator for several days, not only did the antioxidant capacity not go down (as anticipated), but some of the produce's flavonoid content actually increased.

Flavonoids are compounds in fruits and vegetables that give them their colour. They also have antioxidant properties. Which means that storing your fruits and vegetables for a few days before you eat them could be a simple way to boost your antioxidant intake – and, in turn, help ward off all the problems that come along with the free radical damage those antioxidants fight: conditions like cancer and heart disease and even things like skin wrinkling and other signs of ageing.

And if this research looks promising for 'regular' fruits and vegetables, imagine how a few days' storage could affect organic produce, which already has a nutritional leg-up on commercially grown varieties thanks to an absence of pesticides and herbicides. For more information on the benefits of choosing organic, see page 201.

But whatever type of fruit and veg you buy, this is something you can do right away, and it won't cost you an extra penny – always a winning combination when it comes to health advice.

A good way of including more fruits in your diet is to juice them in a blender. Try adding sliced fruit to your cereal too, which is both delicious and healthy.

The following fruits have been selected for the remarkable health benefits they deliver. However, don't limit yourself to eating these fruits alone, as all fruits have their own unique therapeutic properties and, once again, 'variety' really is the key to taking advantage of all they have to offer.

Açaí: Nature's perfect food – the amazing health benefits of the fruit from the Amazon's 'tree of life'

A super food from the Amazon, fresh from the tree, provides over 30 times the amount of anthocyanins (potent antioxidants) as red wine and all the beneficial fatty acids of olive oil in one delicious, all-natural package. And this is just the beginning of this food's health benefits. It's virtually impossible to overdo this food – which is certainly not the case with red wine or olive oil.

There's no disputing the health benefits of anthocyanins and essential fatty acids. Both have proven to be powerful nutritional tools in the quest for good health. The cardiovascular benefits of anthocyanins are the most well known; studies show that they can help prevent blood clots, improve blood circulation, relax blood vessels and prevent atherosclerosis (*Bratisl Lek Listy 2002; 103(4-5): 159-165; FASEB J 2002 Dec;16(14):1958-1960*). But scientists have also discovered that they possess powerful antiviral and anti-allergenic properties. Some research even suggests that they can prevent cancer and encourage tumour cell death (*Curr Mol Med 2003 Mar; 3(2): 149-159*).

Essential fatty acids have proven just as powerful. Oleic acid, a monounsaturated omega-9 acid, and linoleic acid, a polyunsaturated omega-6 acid, help lower LDL ('bad' cholesterol) levels and maintain HDL ('good' cholesterol) levels. They also increase the absorption of fat-soluble vitamins like vitamins A, E, D, and K, which are essential to good health. Research has even suggested that oleic acid may prevent against cancer and hypertension (*J Lipid Res 2003 Mar; 44(3): 567-575*).

Olive oil may be the best known source of these nutrients, but it is certainly not the only one. It's the pigment in red grapes that gives wine its anthocyanins – and that same pigment can also be found in other red and purple fruits and vegetables, such as blueberries, red cabbage and purple sweet potatoes.

Oleic acid is also present in pecans and seed oils, and linoleic acid is found in peanuts. But there is one food that delivers it all – plus other healthy nutrients like fibre, phytosterols, and vitamins C and E. For centuries, it's been a staple for people in Brazil, yet virtually unknown to anyone outside the region – until now. It's called açaí (pronounced ah-sigh-ee), and it's the fruit of a palm tree that grows in the rainforests of the Amazon – a tree Brazilians call the 'The Tree of Life'.

Discover the health secret of generations of Amazonian Indians

About 90 per cent of the small, round fruit consists of açaí's hard, inedible pit – but that's not a problem, because it's the outside skin that holds the treasure. The dark purple skin is what contains the anthocyanins.

The natives purée the skins, creating a treat that can be served warm as a sauce over fruit or grains, or frozen like a sorbet. They've been eating it for centuries, passing down recipes from generation to generation. Because the fruit itself is perishable, its popularity never spread beyond the region.

Then, a few years ago, two friends from California went to Brazil on a surfing expedition and tasted açaí for the first time. Before they even knew the health benefits, they were hooked on the taste. But once they learned that the tasty treat was also a nutritional powerhouse, they knew they had to find a way to bring açaí to the rest of the world.

Super food fights heart disease, cancer, prostate enlargement and more

Since then, the news about açaí has been steadily spreading – and the evidence of nutritional and health benefits just keep piling up. Consider this: a 100-gram serving of açaí contains only 90 calories, just two grams of fat and no cholesterol. Plus, it delivers 3.5 grams of dietary fibre, something we could all use more of in our diets as you'll discover on page 92.

Improved processing of the fresh fruit is making it possible to preserve more of the fruit's healthful attributes. Currently, the purée provides more anthocyanins than red wine and has antioxidant concentrations that well outweigh blueberries. Subsequent research has shown that in addition to anthocyanins and essential fatty acids, açaí also contains a healthy dose of plant sterols, another class of phytochemicals that have been shown to reduce cholesterol, protect the immune system, and relieve prostate enlargement (*Life Sci 2000 Jun 30; 67(6): 605-615*).

In fact, it turns out açaí is in the same family as saw palmetto, a common herbal treatment for prostate enlargement. And researchers at the Federal University of Rio de Janeiro have discovered that açaí extract can be used to fight infection, like the common bacterial infection *Staphylococcus aureus*. It seems there's no end to this miracle fruit's health benefits.

What to take for best results

Although açaí may not be available in your local supermarket, you can find it in several health food and gourmet stores (often in juice form).

Refreshing açaí and mango smoothie

This drink serves 1 person

For this drink you will need the following ingredients:

50g açaí berry pulp
50g mango
150g apple juice
2 strawberries

To Prepare:

Simply mix all the ingredients in a blender, pour into a glass and drink. Enjoy!

An apple a day really can help keep your doctor away...

There are many benefits linked to eating apples. For example, numerous studies have shown that eating them on a regular basis can help reduce the risk of cancer:

- quercetin, a flavonoid abundant in apples has been found to help prevent the growth of prostate cancer cells
- Phytonutrients in the skin of apples are able to inhibit the growth of colon cancer cells by 43 per cent
- Food containing flavonoids, like those in apples, may reduce the risk of lung cancer by as much as 50 per cent
- Dietary phenolics such as flavonoids (found in apples) have inhibitory effects on the developments of carcinogenic substances in the bladder, thereby reducing risk of bladder cancer, especially in smokers

In addition, research has shown that eating apples may help prevent asthma, COPD (a congestive lung condition), and diabetes. In fact, in an October 2005 study, women who ate one apple per day reduced their Type 2 diabetes risk by 28 per cent. Apples, therefore, qualify as an especially good fruit choice for those prone to asthma, bronchitis, or high blood sugar levels.

Studies have shown that a diet rich in apples could help to lower blood cholesterol levels too. Pectin, a soluble fibre found in apples has been thought to play a significant role in this. In fact, apple juice has been found to inhibit the oxidation of the harmful form of cholesterol (LDL, or low-density lipoprotein).

French researchers have found that a flavonoid called phloridzin, which is found only in apples, may protect postmenopausal women from osteoporosis and may also increase bone density. Boron, another ingredient in apples, also strengthens bones.

Besides therapeutic benefits, apples are also found to play a role in inhibiting age-related problems, preventing wrinkles and promoting hair growth (due to a compound named procyanidin B-2).

Apples are great if you're trying to lose weight too as they're a good source of dietary fibre and help to aid digestion and promote weight loss. A 2003 Brazilian study showed that eating three apples a day for 12 weeks helped participants lower their blood-glucose levels and lose an average of 2.7 pounds.

When choosing apples, you're better off buying organic ones in season from local farmers. While you should opt for organic fruits and vegetables whenever possible in general, this advice especially holds true when it comes to apples.

This is because they usually rank among the 12 top fruits and vegetables contaminated by pesticides in tests run by the non-profit Environmental Working Group (EWG), which investigates environmental threats to health. Others on the list include bell peppers, celery, cherries, imported grapes, nectarines, peaches, pears, potatoes, raspberries, spinach and strawberries. The last EWG report on pesticides in fruits and vegetables concluded that frequently eating these 'dirty dozen' will expose a person to about 14 pesticides per day, on average.

In contrast, the 12 least chemically treated fruit and vegetables on the list include: asparagus, avocados, bananas, broccoli, cauliflower, corn (sweet), kiwi, mangos, onions, papaya, pineapples, and peas (sweet).

Pork chops with apple sauce

This recipe serves 4 people

For this dish you will need the following ingredients:

2-3 cooking apples, depending on size (Bramley's are good)
Grated zest of lemon
2 tsp sugar
3 tbsp apple juice
4 pork chops
salt and freshly ground black pepper
4 sage leaves, finely chopped

To prepare:

Peel and core the apples and cut into chunks. Place in a medium saucepan along with the lemon zest, sugar and apple juice. Cover and cook over a very low heat, checking and stirring occasionally until soft, about 10 minutes.

Meanwhile, heat the grill, season the chops and grill for about five minutes each side until done.

Stir the chopped sage into the apple sauce and serve with the pork chops.

Tip: Apple sauce freezes well so you can make a large batch and freeze in small portions for other meals.

How diet remains one of the number 1 antidotes to the ageing process

The latest research offers good news for all of us looking for simple ways to maximize our chances of living a long and healthy life. Researchers in Spain recently found that men and women who consumed a greater amount of fruits, vegetables and antioxidant nutrients experienced fewer deaths during a 6.5 year period (*American Journal of Clinical Nutrition, June 2007*).

Antonio Agudo, of The Catalan Institute of Oncology in Spain, and his fellow researchers, evaluated data from 41,358 Spanish participants in the European Prospective Investigation into Cancer and Nutrition study. Information on diet obtained during interviews was analyzed for alpha-carotene, beta-carotene, beta-cryptoxanthin, lycopene, vitamin C and vitamin E levels. Vegetable intake was grouped and analyzed in five categories, and fresh fruit was analyzed separately from total fruit consumption.

Over the 6.5 year follow-up, 562 deaths occurred among the participants, whose ages ranged between 30 and 69. Participants whose fresh fruit intake was in the top 25 per cent of participants experienced a 21 per cent lower risk of dying than those whose intake was in the lowest fourth. Root vegetable intake in the top fourth was associated with a 28 per cent lower mortality risk, and seed-containing vegetables with a 23 per cent lower risk, compared with those whose intake was lowest.

When antioxidants were examined, lycopene (high amounts of which are present in tomatoes and watermelon – for more details see the section on tomatoes on page 48) intake was associated with the greatest reduction in the risk of death. Subjects whose lycopene intake levels were in the top fourth had a 35 per cent lower risk of death during follow-up compared with men and women whose intake was in the bottom fourth. Vitamin C and carotenoids also appeared to be protective, however, adjustment for total antioxidant capacity in plant foods cancelled the effect.

Commenting on the findings the researchers said: "A high intake of fresh fruit, root vegetables, and fruiting vegetables is associated with reduced mortality, probably as a result of their high content of vitamin C, provitamin A carotenoids and lycopene. Antioxidant capacity could partly explain the effect of ascorbic acid and provitamin A but not the association with lycopene."

Research findings uncover cancer-fighting properties linked to avocados

Avocados are considered by many to be an almost complete food. This is hardly surprising given that they are a rich source of vitamins, minerals and phytonutrients, providing 4 per cent of the recommended Daily Value (DV) for vitamin E, 4 per cent vitamin C, 8 per cent folate, 4 per cent fibre, 2 per cent iron, 4 per cent potassium, with 81mcg of lutein and 19mcg of beta-carotene. They are renowned for their cholesterol-lowering properties and ability to maintain cardiovascular health.

According to the latest research findings from Dr Steven M. D'Ambrosio and his associates at Ohio State University, in the US, it appears that phytochemicals extracted from the popular Haas avocado are able to destroy oral cancer cells as well as prevent pre-cancerous cells from developing into cancer (*report published online ahead of print in the journal Seminars in Cancer Biology*).

Hass avocados are year-round fruits known for their distinctive bumpy skin that turns from green to purplish-black as they ripen. While there are more than 500 varieties of avocados grown worldwide, Hass avocados are the most readily available at supermarkets nationwide. Similar research has not been conducted on other varieties of avocados as yet, so it is not clear if these benefits are limited to Hass avocados alone or extend to all types.

For the purpose of this study, Dr D'Ambrosio, who is a member of the molecular carcinogenesis and chemoprevention program at OSU's Comprehensive Cancer Center, collaborated with Haiming Ding of the Department of Radiology, Young-Won Chin of the College of Pharmacy, and A. Douglas Kinghorn, also of the Comprehensive Cancer Center. They determined that the avocado compounds target multiple signalling pathways and increase intracellular reactive oxygen in pre-cancerous cells to trigger programmed cell death, while leaving healthy cells unharmed.

Commenting on the findings, Dr D'Ambrosio said: "As far as we know, this is the first study of avocados and oral cancer. We think these phytochemicals either stop the growth of pre-cancerous cells in the body or they kill the pre-cancerous cells without affecting normal cells. Our study focuses on oral cancer, but the findings might have implications for other types of cancer. These are preliminary findings, and more research is needed."

He went on to add: "The future is ripe for identifying fruits and vegetables and individual phytonutrients with cancer preventing activity. As we identify the molecular mechanisms and targets by which individual phytonutrients prevent cancer, we may be able to improve upon nature by formulating phytonutrient cocktails for specific cancers and individual susceptibility and risk."

Numerous studies in the past have revealed how a high consumption of fruit and vegetables is linked to a reduced risk of various types of cancer. The protective effect is attributed to the high levels of phytonutrients or phytochemicals – plant compounds thought to have health-protecting qualities – that are often found in dark coloured fruits and vegetables.

Spicy avocado dip to wake up your taste buds

This recipe serves 1-2 people

For this dish you will need the following ingredients:

1 large ripe avocado
1 clove of garlic, peeled and chopped
1 green chilli, chopped
2 ½ oz of unflavoured fromage frais
3 tbsp of fresh coriander leaves

1 tbsp of lemon juice
¼ tsp of salt
¼ tsp of ground cumin
1 large red pepper, sliced into long strips for dipping
1 large carrot, cut into batons for dipping

To prepare:

Slice the avocado into two (length ways) and remove the stone.

Scoop out the flesh and put into a food processor with all the other ingredients except the cumin. Blend well.

Move the dip into its serving dish and sprinkle the cumin over the top.

Simply dip in your carrot and pepper sticks and enjoy!

The bountiful benefits of bananas

Bananas are an excellent source of vitamin B6 and vitamin C, dietary fibre, manganese and potassium. With regards to the latter they really excel and offer one of our best sources of this essential mineral.

Potassium is necessary for maintaining normal blood pressure and heart function. Since the average banana contains a whopping 467mg of potassium and only 1mg of sodium, a banana a day can help to prevent high blood pressure and protect against atherosclerosis.

In addition to these cardiovascular benefits, the potassium found in bananas may also help to promote bone health. Research indicates that potassium may counteract the increased urinary calcium loss caused by a high-salt diet, thus helping to prevent bones from thinning out at a fast rate.

Bananas have also long been recognized for their antacid effects that protect against stomach ulcers and ulcer damage. In one study, a simple mixture of banana and milk significantly suppressed acid secretion. They work their protective magic in two ways:

First, substances in bananas help activate the cells that compose the stomach lining, so they produce a thicker protective mucus barrier against stomach acids. Second, other compounds in bananas called protease inhibitors help eliminate bacteria in the stomach that have been pinpointed as a primary cause of stomach ulcers.

Bananas, like most fibre, tend to help both diarrhoea and constipation. A bout of diarrhoea can quickly deplete your body of important electrolytes. Bananas can replenish your stores of potassium, one of the most vital electrolytes, which helps regulate heart function as well as fluid balance. In addition, bananas contain pectin, a soluble fibre (called a hydrocolloid) that can help normalize movement through the digestive tract and ease constipation.

Bananas are an unusually rich fruit source of protein, and their energising qualities make them a good fruit to have for breakfast. Add chopped bananas and a handful of walnuts to cereal, such as porridge, to give you plenty of get up and go in the mornings.

Paradoxically, besides being energising, bananas contain tryptophan, an amino acid with naturally sedative effects, which makes them a good bedtime snack if you have trouble sleeping. Tryptophan has the additional benefit of being a natural mood enhancer so can help if you suffer from PMT or depression.

Banana and raisin bread

For this dish you will need the following ingredients:

3 bananas
6 oz of raisins

4 oz butter

8 oz self raising flour

4 oz soft brown sugar

2 eggs

2 tbsp honey

To prepare:

Preheat your oven to 180c/350f/Gas Mark 4.

Rub the butter and flour together until breadcrumbs. Next add the sugar and raisins and stir the mixture. Beat in the eggs. Spoon out the honey and stir in. Mash the bananas and add to the mixture and again give the mixture a good stir.

Grease a loaf tin and pour in the mixture. Put in the oven and cook for 1 hour. Check to see if it's cooked after this time by putting in a skewer (if it comes out clean then it's ready). Turn out the bread and leave to cool. Enjoy!

Blueberries can protect your brain cells, beat cystitis and stop cancer in its tracks

With a one-in-three chance of developing cancer in your lifetime, a one-in-two chance of suffering from coronary heart disease and a high probability you will suffer some form of age-related brain damage, you are naturally committed to taking an active role in your own health. And there is a simple fruit that can help you fight, not one, but all three of these modern scourges – and tackle other problems such as cystitis and poor liver function too!

Scientists have known for some time that all dark coloured berries are packed full of beneficial plant chemicals. What they didn't know until recently was that one particular type of berry is way ahead of the others, in terms of its antioxidant and anti-ageing chemical contents. This type of berry is the wild blueberry (*Vaccinium angustifolium*).

In a survey of 22 different fruits and vegetables, blueberries came top regarding antioxidant content (*J Agric Food Chem 1996, 44: 701-705*). They contained more antioxidants than garlic, spinach, strawberries, broccoli or kale, which are themselves rich sources of antioxidants.

A particular form of antioxidants found to be highly concentrated in wild blueberries is anthocyanins – plant chemicals able to fight heart disease, cancer and ageing (*J Agric Food Chem 1998, 46: 2686-2693*).

Researchers studying blueberries' enormous range of health benefits found that, although blueberries consumed in processed form contain powerful antioxidants, eating raw berries gives you the full benefits of their ingredients. This is because food processing and exposure to heat reduces the antioxidant content of the fruit.

But the humble blueberry has many more powerful components in its arsenal against ageing. Other highly efficient antioxidants found in blueberry extracts are ascorbic acid (vitamin C), the plant agents called tannins (tea is another rich source of tannins too!), and quercetin – a chemical that protects against heart disease by preventing blood from abnormal clotting in the arteries. Blueberries are so rich in beneficial natural chemicals that half a cup of wild blueberries is equivalent to two or three cups of other berries!

Avoid harmful repeat antibiotic prescriptions to beat cystitis

Over 50 per cent of women suffer from cystitis at least once in their lives – and many have repeat bouts of this excruciatingly painful condition. Blueberries, like cranberries, are effective in reducing the symptoms of cystitis, such as irritation, burning, and feeling the need to pass urine frequently.

They work by protecting the wall of your bladder, making it impossible for bacteria such as E. coli to attach themselves (*New Eng J Med 1998, 339: 1085-1086*). Consider taking blueberry juice or blueberry extracts in tablet form to prevent and cure urinary infections. You'll avoid the dangers of repeat prescriptions for antibiotics that may cause stomach upset, rashes, nausea or thrush.

Other benefits linked to blueberries:

- Blueberry extract improves liver function. Its ingredients help maintain the liver enzymes in good condition.
- Maintenance of vision, and particularly night vision. Blueberries provide protection to the different sensors within the eye that are responsible for initiating the process of vision.
- Heart disease. Their antioxidant actions shield the muscle tissues of the heart and reduce the process of lipid peroxidation, thus reducing the risk of thickening of the arteries.

The secret of blueberry's four-pronged attack on cancer

Most antioxidants can influence cancer growth and the ingredients in blueberries are particularly effective in stopping cancer growth on several fronts (*J Food Sci 2000, 65: 352-356*):

- They discourage cancer cells from appearing in the first place, through a mechanism as yet to be fully researched.
- They shield healthy cells against injury by deactivating the free radicals produced by abnormal, cancerous cells.
- They block the formation of new blood vessels, which are needed by the fast-growing cancer cells, and so starve these cells of nutrients.
- They boost the immune system, which, in turn, attacks existing cancer cells and eliminates them.

Reverse age-related brain damage with blueberry extracts

Recent research has also discovered that blueberry extracts are able to reverse age-related brain damage in certain cases. The antioxidant activities of blueberries protect brain cells against environmental toxins and free radicals created during your body's normal metabolic processes.

In non-human trials, scientists found that a high consumption of blueberry extracts led to a striking improvement in brain function. Benefits ranged from improvement of the sense of balance, coordination, ability to grasp, memory, learning and resistance to fatigue. All these skills generally worsen with age, but in this experiment, blueberry extracts were shown to actually reverse this decline (*J Neurosci 1999, 19(18) 8114-8121*).

In addition, brain cells may become less stable with age, losing the strength of their membrane, which results in cells filling up with water and eventually dying. This can manifest in memory problems, loss of concentration and inability to process information.

Blueberry extracts protect against this, by strengthening the outside membrane of the cell. Other fruits and vegetables, such as strawberries or spinach, although effective in improving age-related brain changes, are not as effective as blueberries (*J Neurosci 1998 10: 8047-8055*).

Researchers found that blueberry extracts improve the concentration of the chemical dopamine in the brain. Dopamine is low in patients with Parkinson's disease, and this low concentration is also blamed for causing memory problems in older people in general (*Neutr Neurosci 2000 3: 383-397*).

Mouthwatering blueberry muffins

This recipe serves 12 people

For this dish you will need the following ingredients:

150g plain flour
150g stoneground wholemeal bread flour
1 tbsp baking powder
75g caster sugar
1 large size egg
300ml milk
2 tbsp lemon juice
90ml soya oil
125g punnet blueberries

To prepare:

Preheat the oven to 200C, 400F, Gas Mark 6. Mix together the flours, baking powder and sugar in a mixing bowl.

In a jug combine together the egg, milk, lemon juice and oil. Make a well in the centre of the dry ingredients and then gradually mix in the liquid until all the ingredients are almost combined. Add the blueberries and quickly mix in, (the mixture should have a rough looking appearance – over mixing will cause the muffins to go tough).

Lightly oil a 12 hole deep muffin tin, ⅔ fill each hole. Cook for 20-25 minutes, or until golden brown. Allow to cool, then run a palate knife around and remove from the tin. Serve immediately.

For another tasty and simple way to benefit from blueberries see the 'Berry bliss smoothie' recipe on page 47.

Cherries provide a vital defence against Type 2 diabetes and cardiovascular disease

Tart cherries have been found to be beneficial for helping to alleviate gout and other forms of arthritis, including both osteo- and rheumatoid arthritis.

Now, the latest exciting research findings from the US suggest that adding tart cherries to the diet may lower cholesterol, lead to less fat storage and improve antioxidant defences.

While these findings were based on an animal study, and more research is certainly needed to establish whether the same results could expect to be seen in humans, it has important implications for treating metabolic syndrome – a condition characterised by central obesity, hypertension, and disturbed glucose and insulin metabolism. The syndrome, which affects 15 per cent of adult Europeans, has been linked to increased risks of both Type 2 diabetes and cardiovascular disease.

The results, presented by researchers at Experimental Biology 2007 in Washington, D.C., showed that the antioxidant-rich cherries achieved significant health improvements at relatively low levels that could easily be achieved in the human diet.

The study involved 48 male Dahl Salt-Sensitive rats – a strain of rats susceptible to salt-linked high blood pressure, high cholesterol and impaired glucose tolerance – which were fed a carbohydrate-enriched diet or a diet that, by weight, included one or 10 per cent cherries for 90 days.

Lead researcher E. Mitcell Seymour and his co-workers, from the University of Michigan Health System, found that both cherry-supplemented groups had significantly lower levels of total cholesterol, triglyceride (blood fat), glucose and insulin than those of the rats that did not receive the cherries.

Plasma antioxidant levels also increased, as measured by Trolox equivalent antioxidant capacity (TEAC). The rats that received cherries had higher antioxidant capacity, indicating lower oxidative stress in their bodies, than those that did not, said the researchers. No toxic effects were observed for either of the cherry doses.

Commenting on the findings, Seymour said: "Rats fed tart cherries as one per cent of their total diet had reduced markers of metabolic syndrome. Previous research by other groups studied pure anthocyanin [antioxidants that give the fruit its bright red hue] compounds rather than anthocyanin-containing wholefoods, and they used concentrations of anthocyanins that would be very difficult if not impossible to obtain in the diet. We are enthusiastic about the findings that tart cherries conferred these beneficial effects at such a modest daily intake."

The researchers' work is ongoing, with studies now being carried out in animals prone to both obesity and diabetes. Additionally, a team of US researchers from the University of Michigan is reported to be launching a small clinical trial to investigate if similar findings are achievable in humans.

Fight muscle pain following exercise simply by drinking cherry juice

The health benefits of exercise – from warding off depression to helping maintain a healthy heart – is hardly ground-breaking news. However, the 'no pain, no gain' aspect of exercise can be enough to put off even the most well-intentioned of us.

The good news is that a recent study published online in the *British Journal of Sports* has revealed that exercise-induced muscle pain could soon become a thing of the past simply by drinking cherry juice.

In light of the numerous antioxidant and anti-inflammatory properties cherries contain, a research team headed by Professor Declan Connolly, of the University of Vermont, evaluated the efficacy of a tart cherry juice blend in preventing the symptoms of muscle damage in a randomised, placebo-controlled study involving 14 male college students.

The study participants were asked to either drink a bottle of the cherry juice blend twice a day for three days before exercise and for four days afterwards, or to drink a placebo juice containing no cherries. The 12-ounce bottle of juice contained the liquid equivalent of 50 to 60 tart cherries blended with commercially available apple juice.

The participants performed a type of strenuous arm muscle exercise – flexing and tensing one arm 20 times – that creates contractions in which the muscle is lengthened. Muscle tenderness, motion and strength were assessed on each of the days before and after exercise, using standard pieces of equipment designed for this purpose. In addition, the study participants rated their muscle soreness on a scale of one to 10. The whole process was repeated all over again two weeks later, with those who had taken the placebo juice taking the cherry juice blend instead, and vice versa. The other arm was also used.

There was a significant difference in the degree of muscle strength loss between those drinking the cherry juice blend and those taking the placebo juice. Muscle strength among subjects who received the placebo fell by 22 per cent, but by only four per cent in those drinking the cherry juice. Participants who received the cherry juice also reported improvement in muscle strength 96 hours after exercising, and less pain. The highest pain scores in the cherry juice drinkers occurred 24 hours following exercise, while among those who received the placebo, pain increased for 48 hours.

Commenting on the study, professor Declan Connelly said: "The anti-inflammatory properties of cherry juice have been examined before, but the focus of this research was on a new area – muscle damage repair."

He went on to say: "These results have important practical applications for athletes, as performance after damaging exercise bouts is primarily affected by strength loss and pain."

Let's hope the current study now paves the way for more research into the potential health benefits of cherry juice.

Cherry sorbet – for the occasional tasty treat

This recipe serves 6 people

For this dish you will need the following ingredients:

1.5kg/3lb cherries
600g/20 oz caster sugar
250ml/8fl oz water
The juice of 1 lemon
1 vanilla pod, split in half lengthwise

Wash and pat dry the cherries. Remove the stones. Place the flesh in a food processor and purée until smooth. Set aside. Place the sugar and water in a heavy based saucepan. Add the vanilla and place over a low to medium heat. Once the sugar has dissolved turn up the heat slightly and simmer for 3-4 minutes or until the syrup feels slightly viscous between your fingers.

Remove from the stove and allow to cool completely. When cool, remove the vanilla pod and pour over the puréed cherries. Squeeze over the lemon juice and stir to combine. Pour into a freezer-proof container and mix the sorbet regularly with a fork as it freezes, or process it in a food processor once frozen.

Cranberries can help fight antibiotic-resistant urinary tract infections

Research has revealed that cranberries provide important protection to the urinary tract from antibiotic-resistant bacteria – in particular the bacterium Escherichia coli. Antibiotic resistance occurs when bacteria develop immunity to common drugs used to combat them – meaning that they become ineffective and fail to treat the condition they've been prescribed to treat. Another drawback to antibiotics is that even when they do work, they kill beneficial bacteria in your body as well as destroying harmful bacteria.

US scientists from Rutgers University and the University of Michigan who conducted the study, isolated Escherichia coli from the urine of women diagnosed with urinary tract infections (UTIs). They then transferred the E. coli bacterium into urine samples collected from healthy participants, before and after they were given eight ounces of cranberry juice.

When the bacteria were introduced into the samples taken before cranberry juice was administered, bacteria stuck to urinary tract cells. In the samples taken after the cranberry juice was consumed, 79 per cent of antibiotic resistant bacteria failed to adhere to the cells.

The beneficial component of cranberries appears to be their proanthocyanidins, which prevent certain E. coli bacteria from adhering to the urinary tract. The researchers concluded that regular consumption of cranberry juice may help reduce the incidence of urinary tract infections and the need for antibiotics.

Study co-author and Professor of Epidemiology at the University of Michigan School of Public Health, Betsy Foxman, commented: "In light of the increasing antibiotic resistance of many bacteria, the public health significance of the role of foods, such as cranberry juice cocktail, in preventing infections warrants further consideration... Additional work that I co-authored, cited in the October 4, 2001 edition of *The New England Journal of Medicine*, suggests that an increasing number of new E. coli strains are resistant to the most common antibiotics used to treat UTIs, prompting physicians and researchers to look for alternatives."

Cranberries offer vital protection in the fight against heart disease

New research findings suggest that cranberries may help to lower the risk of heart disease too.

At the recent 225th national meeting of the American Chemical Society, Professor Joe Vinson from the University of Scranton in the US, reported on how daily consumption of cranberry juice was able to raise high-density lipoprotein (HDL) levels – 'good' cholesterol – by 10 per cent. This provides a corresponding decrease in heart disease risk of 40 per cent.

The US study involved 19 patients suffering from elevated cholesterol levels. They received blood tests at the study's onset and then each month for a period of three months in total. The participants were given one eight ounce glass of cranberry juice each day for one month, followed by two glasses for the second month and three glasses per day for the concluding month of the study.

The researchers also found that antioxidant levels in the participants' blood increased by more than 120 per cent, after they received two or more servings of cranberry juice daily. Increased antioxidants are strongly associated with lower heart disease risk.

According to the researchers, cranberries' benefits for lowering cholesterol levels and heart disease risk are probably due to the high levels of polyphenols they contain. Polyphenols are natural plant chemicals that possess a potent antioxidant effect. Of 20 commonly consumed fruits, cranberries have been shown to be among those with the highest levels of polyphenols.

Lead researcher of the study, Dr Vinson, stated: "This study gives consumers another reason to consider drinking cranberry juice, which has more health benefits than previously believed. People should consider drinking it with their meals."

Prevent tooth decay and plaque build-up with cranberries

Cranberries really are proving their worth as a super fruit. Scientists have discovered that the flavonoids quercetin and myricetin found in cranberries can also stop the formation of dental plaque and tooth decay.

This is promising news as tooth decay is said to be the most common oral infection, with over 95 per cent of all adults having experienced it. It results from the interaction of specific bacteria with constituents of the diet on a susceptible tooth surface.

Dental plaque accumulation is the first evidence of this interaction; dental plaque is a biofilm that is comprised of bacteria that grow on the tooth surface. Acid can be formed rapidly by acidogenic bacteria, such as Streptococcus mutans, and its presence eventually results in the decay of the tooth.

Past research has shown that cranberries are able to prevent the adhesion of Streptococcus mutans to teeth.

The new research, presented recently at the 84th General Session of the International Association for Dental Research, goes some way to identifying the compounds in cranberries that could be responsible for this benefit.

US scientists from the University of Rochester School of Medicine and Dentistry in New York reported that flavonoids in cranberries might be able to prevent tooth decay by reducing the formation of plaque, inhibiting acidic conditions, and preventing harmful bacteria from sticking to teeth.

Previous research from the same scientists led the British Dental Health Foundation, which offers impartial dental advice to the public, to advise people to drink cranberry juice (in moderation and at mealtimes) to boost oral health.

Lead researcher Hyun Koo and his colleagues investigated the effects of the flavonoids quercetin and myricetin on the inhibition of glucosyltransferase enzymes (GTF), which are associated with plaque formation. Tests were performed in solution and on saliva-coated hydroxyapatite (calcium compounds sometimes used in dental implants).

They found that solutions containing 250 micrograms per millilitre of the flavonoids quercetin and myricetin inhibited the activity of glucosyltransferase enzymes by about 55 per cent in solution and by as much as 40 per cent on the hydroxyapatite.

In addition, the gene responsible for producing the glucosyltransferase enzymes was found to be repressed. The flavonoids also inhibited the drop in pH (acid conditions) when the bacteria were kept in solution.

Commenting on the findings the researchers said: "Our data show that quercetin and myricetin are active compounds in cranberry that modulate the virulence factors involved in S. mutans acidogenicity and biofilm formation."

Festive cranberry sauce – the perfect accompaniment to turkey

For this dish you will need the following ingredients:

1lb cranberries
Half a pint of water
Half a lb of castor sugar
Grated rind of half a lemon
Sprig of fresh mint

To prepare:

Preheat your oven to 150C/300F/Gas Mark 2.

Place all the ingredients in a small heat-resistant container, cover with a lid or foil, place in the oven and allow to cook until all the cranberry skins are broken. Serve hot or cold sprinkled lightly with chopped fresh mint.

How the health benefits of oranges extend beyond vitamin C

Oranges are one of Mother Nature's best super foods, packed with an unbelievable array of disease-fighting nutrients, all tucked neatly beneath the peel. The fruit has long been known to be a rich source of immune-boosting vitamin C, which plays an important role in cancer prevention, healthy blood circulation and wound healing.

Now, Californian scientists have discovered that oranges are also rich in compounds called citrus limonoids. These chemicals have been proven to help fight a number of varieties of cancer, including that of the mouth, skin, lung, breast, stomach and colon.

The researchers have found that each time we bite into a citrus slice or drink a glass of orange juice, our bodies can readily access a limonoid called limonin, which as well as having cancer-fighting properties can also help lower cholesterol.

Oranges are also rich in the following healthy nutrients:

- Beta-carotene, a powerful antioxidant that protects against cell damage.
- Calcium, which helps protect and maintain the health of your bones and teeth.
- Folic acid which is needed for proper brain development.
- Magnesium for helping maintain blood pressure.
- Potassium, which is necessary for maintaining electrolyte balance in the cells, and is important in maintaining a healthy cardiovascular system.
- Thiamin, which helps to convert food into energy.
- Vitamin B6, which helps support the production of haemoglobin that carries oxygen to all parts of your body.
- Pectin – This water-soluble fibre helps reduce blood cholesterol levels and can aid weight loss by suppressing hunger levels up to four hours after it's eaten.

Orange and lemon roasted chicken

This recipe serves 4 people

For this dish you will need the following ingredients:

1 organic chicken, about 1.63kg (3½lb)
1 large orange, cut into quarters
2 unwaxed lemons, halved
2tbsp extra virgin olive oil
Handful thyme sprigs

To prepare:

Pre-heat your oven to 200C, 400F, Gas Mark 6.

Lay the chicken, breast side down, on a board. Using sharp scissors, cut down either side of the backbone. Turn the chicken over and press to flatten, using the heel of your hand.

Place breast side down in a roasting tray and season well. Drizzle over the olive oil, scatter over the thyme and roast for 30 minutes.

Remove the roasting tin from the oven and reduce the heat to 180C, 350F, Gas Mark 4. Squeeze the juice from the lemons and orange over the chicken, then add the citrus pieces to the tray and turn the chicken over. Roast for a further 30-40 minutes until the chicken is cooked through. To test, pierce the thickest part of the thigh with a skewer; the juices should run clear. If they are pink, return to the oven for a little longer.

Remove the chicken from the oven, cover with foil and leave to rest in a warm place for 10 minutes before carving.

Eat more pineapple to maintain good joint health

The pineapple may sound like an unlikely source of healing powers, but an extract from its stem has been shown to act as an effective natural anti-inflammatory that reduces pain and swelling, improves joint mobility and promotes tissue repair.

In fact, pineapples have been traditionally used as a medicinal plant in parts of the world where the fruit is in abundant supply. In Hawaii, for example, the fruit has long been used by native people as an effective cure for digestive problems and sore throats.

Apart from being a rich source of vitamin C, the pineapple contains an active substance known as bromelain; this is primarily made up of a digestive enzyme but also contains other enzymes, such as peroxidase and acid phosphatase, as well as calcium. It is bromelain, which has been clinically proven to ease joint pain and discomfort.

Research has shown that bromelain is able to inhibit the action of prostaglandins, which cause pain and inflammation, and also helps with the breakdown of fibrin, a protein associated with fluid retention and swelling (*Cohen A, Goldman J. 1964. Bromelain therapy in rheumatoid arthritis. Pennsylvania Med J, 67, 27-30*).

Simple-to-prepare pineapple salsa

This recipe serves 2 people as an accompaniment (tastes delicious with fish)

For this dish you will need the following ingredients:

½ fresh pineapple
½ red pepper
½ red onion (finely chopped)
1 tsp fresh ginger (finely chopped)
2 tbsp lime juice
3 tbsp fresh coriander leaves (chopped)
½ fresh chilli (chopped)

To prepare:

Peel the pineapple and remove all hard cores and 'eyes'. Chop the pineapple and pepper into small cubes and combine well with the remaining ingredients in a bowl. Chill in the fridge until needed.

The remarkable anti-cancer and anti-inflammatory properties linked to pomegranates

There's an excellent reason for all of the hype that's built up around pomegranates. They've been found to reduce inflammation, fight tumour formation, boost heart health, and protect your vision.

Pomegranates are an antioxidant powerhouse, packed with polyphenolic compounds like flavonoids (especially anthocyanins, which give the pulp its rich red colour) and hydrolysable tannins (which can also be found in green tea and red wine). Among the most important polyphenols in pomegranates, though, is a class of tannins called ellagitannins – the compounds responsible for (among other things) the formation of ellagic acid.

Ellagic acid is one of your greatest allies in the fight against cancer. Invitro studies have demonstrated its ability to inhibit the growth of various types of cancer cells (including breast and colon) and to shrink existing tumours by means of apoptosis (programmed cell death) (*J Nutr Biochem. 2004 Nov; 15(11): 672-8*).

But unfortunately, free ellagic acid is of little use in a clinical context, as it demonstrates minimal (if any) antioxidant activity under these conditions. It's virtually unusable to your body in this synthetic form (and may actually result in potentially serious side effects, such as heightened blood pressure).

When bound to glucose in the form of natural ellagitannins, however, its efficacy as a cancer-fighting antioxidant is increased substantially. That's because ellagitannins are extremely water-soluble and bioavailable – and when consumed, your body will synthesize its own ellagic acid as a natural by-product of digestion. This is why fruits that contain these ellagitannins – such as blueberries, strawberries, raspberries... and yes, pomegranates – have assumed a key nutritional role in the prevention and treatment of cancer.

But since every plant has a different phytochemical structure, it's important to note that the most active components of each are bound to differ. In fact, it's actually one particular family of ellagitannins known as punicosides (and specifically punicalagin – both of which are terms derived from the fruit's latin name, *Punica granatum*) that have been pegged as the primary polyphenols at work in pomegranates – not ellagic acid, as once thought (*Eur J Nutr. 2003 Jan; 42(1): 18-28*).

Researchers now recognise that these punicalagins work synergistically with the ellagic acid they help to form in the human body, thereby delivering the results that we've seen in so many studies (*J Nutr Biochem. 2005 Jun; 16(6): 360-7*). And it's this total picture that accounts for pomegranate's demonstrated ability to (among other things) fight tumours.

Attention all men – pomegranates can benefit your love life and prostate health

US researchers from The Male Clinic, Beverly Hills, and University of California, Los Angeles, have found that drinking a glass of pomegranate juice every day may help manage erectile dysfunction (ED) (*International Journal of Impotence Research (Nature Publishing) Advance online publication 14 June 2007; doi: 10.1038/sj.ijir.3901570*).

The researchers assigned 61 male subjects suffering from mild to moderate erectile dysfunction to two four-week intervention periods, separated by a two-week washout. Subjects were assigned to receive either daily pomegranate juice (POM Wonderful, 237ml), or a placebo beverage. Measures of erectile performance were obtained using International Index of Erectile Function (IIEF) and Global

Assessment Questionnaires (GAQ).

At the end of the randomised, placebo-controlled, double-blind, crossover pilot study, 47 per cent of the subjects reported erection improvements after consuming the pomegranate juice, while only 32 per cent reported improvements during the placebo phase.

Commenting on the findings the researchers said: "Subjects were more likely to have improved scores when pomegranate juice was consumed. Although overall statistical significance was not achieved, this pilot study suggests the possibility that larger cohorts and longer treatment periods may achieve statistical significance."

The researchers believe that the beneficial results might be due to the potent antioxidant content of pomegranate juice, which can prevent free radical molecules from disrupting proper circulatory function.

Pomegranate's benefits for men's health don't end there...

Pomegranate juice may benefit men's health in another way too, as research suggests that it helps prevent the progression of prostate cancer (*J Nutr Biochem. 2004 Nov; 15 (11): 672-8*). In fact, US researchers from the University of California in Los Angeles say the effect may be so large that it may help older men outlive the disease.

The UCLA team focused on 50 men who had undergone surgery or radiation treatment for prostate cancer – but had shown signs that the disease was rapidly returning.

The presence of prostate cancer cells is monitored by measuring levels of a chemical they produce called prostate-specific antigen (PSA). The researchers measured how long it took for PSA levels to double in individual patients – a short doubling time indicates that the cancer is progressing quickly.

The average doubling time is about 15 months, but in patients who drank pomegranate juice this increased to an average of 54 months. Some men on the study continued to show suppressed PSA levels after more than three years, even though they were receiving no treatment apart from drinking pomegranate juice.

Pomegranates beat apples in the antioxidant stakes

According to the results of a new study, pomegranate juice is more effective than apple juice in boosting the body's antioxidant defences, which naturally decline with age (*Nutrition Research (Elsevier), February 2008, Volume 28, Issue 2, Pages 72-77*).

Researchers from the Institute of Hygiene and Environmental Medicine in Tianjin, China, found that the antioxidant capacity of the blood of 26 elderly subjects increased by almost 10 per cent after drinking pomegranate juice, whereas changes were negligible after drinking apple juice.

Pomegranate, known as the royal fruit because of the 'crown' on top, is a rich source of antioxidants. It is these antioxidants, and particularly ellagitannin compounds like punicalagins and punicalins, which accounts for about half of the fruit's antioxidant ability.

Indeed, according to the researchers, it is these compounds which most likely account for boosting the antioxidant capacity of the elderly subjects in the new study.

Lead researcher Changjiang Guo said: "Because the plasma ascorbic acid, vitamin E, and reduced glutathione contents did not differ significantly between the two groups in this study, the phenolics may be the functional components contained in pomegranate juice that accounted for the observations."

For the purpose of the study the subjects (average age 63.5) were

---

randomly divided into two groups and assigned to drink 250ml daily of either apple or pomegranate juice for four weeks.

At the end of the study the researchers found that the plasma antioxidant capacity of the subjects consuming pomegranate juice had increased from 1.33 to 1.46 millimoles per litre (mmol/l), using the FRAP assay of antioxidant quantification. On the other hand, the antioxidant capacity of the subjects consuming apple juice changed negligibly from 1.37 to 1.36 mmol/l.

Furthermore, urine levels of 8-hydroxydeoxyguanosine (8-OH-dG), the product of hydroxyl radical attack – reportedly a marker of damaged DNA – was reduced by about 21 per cent more in the pomegranate group than in the apple group, report the researchers. However, they failed to detect significant changes in cellular DNA damage. DNA damage from oxidative stress has been linked to an increased risk of various diseases, particularly cancer.

Processing makes (almost) perfect

There's no doubting the health benefits a daily dose of pomegranates can provide. And when it comes down to a choice between eating the fruit and drinking its juice, you might expect that the first of these two would be the better option – fruit is almost always healthier for you than juice alone, thanks to the extra bit of fibre that comes with it.

But this is one of those rare cases when, unless you plan to eat the entire pomegranate (rind and all), you're actually better off going with the juice – that is, assuming that it's commercially prepared.

One study published in the *Journal of Agricultural and Food Chemistry* showed that commercially prepared juice has higher antioxidant activity than home-made juices obtained from the arils (sacks of pulp) alone.

Further analysis revealed that commercial juices contained substantial amounts of punicalagin, while the juice prepared from the arils showed only trace amounts of this ellagitannin. The researchers concluded that additional hydrolysable tannins in the pomegranate's skin are extracted during commercial processing (*J Agric Food Chem. 2000 Oct; 48(10): 4581-9*).

None of this is to say, of course, that there's no benefit in eating pomegranate, or drinking juice that you've prepared for yourself – it simply means that eating the entire fruit is the only way to prevent perfectly good polyphenols from going to waste.

Besides, most of the studies that confirm the healing powers of pomegranate are based around the fruit's juice anyway – so all in all, one cup of pure pomegranate juice a day is probably the most reliable form of this antioxidant that you can get. Nevertheless, there's a major drawback to this mode of delivery: the juice's natural sugar and calorie content.

One eight-ounce glass will set you back a substantial 160 calories and 34 grams of sugar. And while in the grand scheme of things this may seem like a fair trade, the compromise is far more problematic if you're diabetic. In this case, your best bet is to opt for pomegranate in supplement form instead.

Pomegranate supplements – know what to look for on the label

Make sure you find a supplement made from whole pomegranates, as opposed to an ellagic acid extract – a tip that makes a lot of sense based on what we've already said about synthetic versions of this polyphenol.

For this same reason, a supplement containing a complete

ellagitannin complex is far more desirable than one containing additional ellagic acid that has already been synthesized in a laboratory – as this could degrade the effectiveness of the pomegranate supplement overall.

All of this also suggests, of course, that you probably shouldn't buy a product that is standardised to a percentage of ellagic acid. While it is indeed an important aspect of pomegranate's antioxidant profile, it's only in the greater context of the fruit's total punicosides (such as in the form of juice, or a whole-fruit extract) that its presence is noteworthy in a supplement (*J Med Food. 2006 Spring; 9(1): 119-22*). So, look for a product that is standardized to these punicosides instead.

You'll also find a lot of products on the market that include pomegranate as part of a long list of ingredients. But watch out as it's not uncommon for manufacturers to pass off deceptively small amounts of any given ingredient in the guise of their own 'proprietary blend'.

The bottom line: Be wary of any pomegranate formula that doesn't list the exact amount of extract present in each dosage on the label, because you might not be getting much of the good stuff at all.

The dark purple smoothie loaded with antioxidants

This drink serves 1 person

For this drink you will need the following ingredients:

125ml pomegranate juice
250ml frozen mixed berries
60ml probiotic vanilla yoghurt
½ tsp cinnamon

To prepare:

Simply put all the ingredients in a blender for 20 seconds or until smooth. Pour into a glass and drink (be careful as this purple mixture can stain your clothes).

Raspberries offer a simple way to protect against cancer

After nearly a decade of research, US physician Dr Daniel W. Nixon of the Hollings Cancer Center in Charleston, South Carolina, has concluded that a substance found in raspberries can help the body purge itself of pre-cancerous growths and even kill existing cancer cells. While no one is suggesting that this simple berry is a miracle cure it could help your immune system fight off the disease.

As far back as 1989, laboratory tests concluded that ellagic acid, which the digestive system extracts from a plant constituent called ellagitannins, can both prevent cancer and kill existing cancer cells (*Planta Med. 1989 Apr; 55(2): 117-22*).

Nixon recognised the potential of ellagic acid and has spent the last eight years researching its benefits, including how to maximise its effects. He discovered that one of the keys to its effectiveness lies in how the substance is ingested.

Nixon discovered that raspberries – specifically the seeds – are a particularly rich source of ellagitannins. He also found that if the seeds are crushed, the digestive system will extract the maximum amount of ellagitannins and create the maximum possible ellagic acid. Additional research shows there's more to raspberries than just the seeds. Both laboratory and animal tests indicate that an even greater cancer killing effect can be achieved when the entire berry is used, especially in puréed form.

Raspberry purée fights cancer in a different way than most other anti-cancer agents – both natural and pharmaceutical. Rather than attacking cancer cells, it stimulates your body's natural immune defences by bolstering a process called the G1 arrest cycle and by increasing p53 gene activity – both of which help stop the spread of mutant cells, including cervical cancer cells (*Cancer Lett, 136(2): 215-21, 1999*). Cells become potentially cancerous when they mutate, and that mutation prevents old, deteriorating cells from dying naturally.

There are a few ways you can tap into the benefits of raspberries. Eat one cup per day (the equivalent of approximately 40mg of ellagitannins). Puréeing the berries is an excellent way to break open the seeds and expose the ellagitannins for better absorption by your digestive system – so add a handful to a blender to make a healthy and delicious smoothie.

Berry bliss smoothie

This recipe serves 2 people

8 strawberries
2 heaped tbsp of raspberries
2 heaped tbsp of blueberries
1 banana
2 glasses of fresh orange juice
2 ice cubes

To prepare:

Place the ingredients in a blender and blend for a good 20 seconds or until the mixture is smooth. Then simply pour into two glasses and drink.

Tomatoes – Why tomato sauce could protect men from prostate cancer

Tomatoes, which scientifically speaking are considered a fruit, deserve a special mention as many scientists believe that a high consumption of tomatoes is linked to a lowered risk of prostate cancer. And now, recent research findings are supporting this belief, and indicate that tomatoes have the ability, not only to prevent prostate cancer, but also to slow down existing cases of the disease.

The naturally-occurring phytochemical, lycopene, which gives tomatoes their red colour, appears to be the key ingredient responsible for this cancer protection. Lycopene is an anti-disease compound, which blocks free radicals, strengthens the immune system, and may help regulate cancer genes. It is also found in red grapefruit.

Research findings from a US study conducted at the University of Illinois in Chicago, which assessed the effects of lycopene, were announced by scientists at the 222nd National Meeting of the American Chemical Society on 29 August 2001.

Tomato sauce was given to prostate cancer patients who were mainly of African-American descent, every day for three weeks. (Up to 34 per cent more African-Americans are diagnosed with prostate cancer than Caucasians and, more disturbingly, this group are twice as likely to die from the disease). Scientists have speculated that genetics and diet may be largely responsible for this statistic.

In Mediterranean countries, the incidence of prostate cancer is far lower, and this is thought to be because Mediterranean men consume more tomato sauce in their diets, than men in other parts of the world.

At the end of the study, participants were found to have a

significant reduction in DNA damage to prostate cells and white blood cells, as well as lower prostate specific antigen (PSA) levels (the protein which is used as a blood marker to determine an individual's risk of prostate cancer).

The study is the first to link a decrease in human DNA damage with consuming tomato sauce. This is important as DNA damage is an indication of an increased risk of cancer. To take advantage of the potent properties of lycopene, eat more tomatoes, or tomato-based products such as tomato sauce (but not tomato ketchup, which often contains little real tomato). Lightly cook tomatoes in a little oil, which enhances the body's ability to absorb lycopene.

Ratatouille – A traditional, tasty way to benefit from tomatoes

This recipe serves 6-8 people

For this dish you will need the following ingredients:

500g courgettes (cut into 1cm thick slices)
1 large aubergine (cut into 1inch chunks)
1 large onion (chopped)
2 garlic cloves (crushed or chopped)
1 red and 1 green pepper (deseeded and cut into slices)
4 tbsp of extra virgin olive oil
400g can of chopped tomatoes
1 tbsp of tomato purée
½ tsp of sugar
1 tsp of coriander seeds
Salt and pepper
2 tbsp of fresh basil (chopped) to garnish

To prepare:

Heat the oil in a large saucepan and add the garlic and onion. Add the aubergine and peppers, stir and then cover. Cook for 10 minutes over a low heat stirring occasionally. Add the courgettes, tomato purée, tomatoes and sugar and season with salt and pepper. Bring to the boil and then lower the heat and simmer gently (uncovered) for about half an hour – stirring occasionally. Crush the coriander seeds and then add to the saucepan and continue cooking for a further 10 minutes, stirring frequently until the mixture is thick. Add the basil to garnish and serve.

Discover how an Asian plum – relied upon by legendary samurai warriors to boost their stamina and energy levels – could benefit your health

Thanks to their healthy diet and lifestyle, Japanese people tend to live longer than many other cultures, with the average life expectancy being 86 years for women and 79 years for men. Not only do the Japenese live to a ripe old age, but according to the World Health Organization, they can also look forward to an average 75 years of being active and disability-free.

One of the reasons for this is thought to be due to the fact that the Japanese eat about 25 per cent fewer calories than we do in the West, probably due to their diet which is largely based on low calorie, nutrient-rich foods – such as fruits, vegetables, rice, noodles, tofu and broth-based soups – rather than the high fat, calorific items we tend to consume. In addition, most Japanese households continue to eat traditional health-giving foods such as miso, seaweed and ume as part of their staple diet.

Ume is a type of edible Asian plum (*Prunus mume*), which belongs to the Rosaceae family. The ume tree originated in China and was later brought to Japan where it is now widely cultivated for its fruit and flowers. It has a long history of use as a medicinal food. During the Middle Ages, the legendary samurai warriors relied on ume fruit to give them energy and counteract battle fatigue. And in the 1920s, Japanese soldiers and sailors were given ume concentrate to help prevent dysentery and motion sickness.

The plums have also been used to rid the body of toxins and parasites and to alleviate gastro-intestinal conditions such as food poisoning and diarrhoea. The standard Japanese folk remedy for colds and flus is a congee (a type of rice porridge) incorporating ume. In addition, they are also recommended as an antidote for hangovers, which is thought to be linked to the fruit's pyric acid content that enhances the break down of alcohol in the liver.

It's hardly surprising that the fruit has so many medicinal properties as it contains numerous active constituents including oleanolic acid (a triterpenoid), citric acid, malic acid, sitosterol (a plant sterol), beta-carotene, vitamins B1, B2, B3, and C, and the minerals calcium, iron and potassium. The constituent principally responsible for the fruits sour flavour is citric acid, which is extremely antibacterial and explains why the plums were used to prevent and relieve the symptoms of food poisoning.

In Japan ume is consumed as both a juice concenrate and as umeboshi or dried, pickled plums. Ume juice concentrate is produced from unripe green plums that are slowly cooked down so that their active ingredients become concentrated. The resulting thick liquid is usually combined with hot water and honey and taken as a tonic. Some traditional Japanese people still begin the day with one or two of the pickled plums and a mug of green tea.

Ume could help fight everything from heart disease to gastric ulcers

The number of studies that support ume's status as an oriental super food is growing and adding them to a daily diet, say researchers, could offer several health-supporting benefits. For instance, as well as boosting energy levels, they can help strengthen your immune system and improve blood circulation.

One scientific paper revealed that ume juice concentrate improved blood fluidity by minimising platelet clumping (blood stickiness). A compound called mumefural, which is produced during the plum processing, is thought to be responsible for this effect. This finding suggests that ume concentrate could be a potential new agent for protecting the body against cardiovascular disease (*J Agric Food Chem. 1999 Mar; 47(3): 828-31*).

Mumefural is considered one of the most alkalising compounds in nature and as most people tend to eat an acid-forming diet – particularly in the West with our heavy reliance on meat, sugar and processed foods – ume concentrate is an ideal solution for neutralising an over-acidic body state.

British author and Japanese food authority Robbie Swinnerton writes, "Japanese pickled plums have remarkable medicinal qualities. Their powerful acidity has a paradoxical alkalinising effect on the body, neutralising fatigue, stimulating the digestion, and promoting the elimination of toxins. This is the Far Eastern equivalent to both aspirin and apple; not only is it a potent hangover remedy for mornings after; more than that, an umeboshi a day is regarded as the best preventive medicine available."

Several other studies have found that unripe ume extract appears to inhibit the activity of Helicobacter pylori – a bacterium that causes chronic inflammation of the lining of the stomach (*Helicobacter.*

2006 Dec;11(6):589-91). It is also the most common cause of gastric and duodenal ulcers worldwide.

In another study that looked at how different fruit and vegetables might protect the body against nitrosamines (compounds present in various foods which are potentially carcinogenic or cancer-forming), ume was effective in reducing the formation of a particular nitrosamine called N-nitrosodimethylamine (*Food and Chemical Toxicology 2002; 40: 949-957*). Tests also show that ume is a potent source of antioxidants, which help fight cancer-causing free radicals and prevent premature ageing (*Nippon Shokuhin Kagaku Kogaku Kaishi, 1999; 46(12): 792-798*).

Delicious vegetarian sushi rolls

This recipe serves 4 people

For this dish you will need the following ingredients:

8 nori sheets
300g sushi rice
2 tbsp of rice wine vinegar
Thinly sliced sticks of carrot, lightly boiled
Thinly sliced sticks of cucumber
Spring onions thinly sliced
Umeboshi plum paste (available from specialist Japanese grocers)
Soy sauce

To Prepare:

Cook the rice as per the instructions on the packet. Add the rice wine vinegar and fluff up with a fork. Leave to cool.

Lay out your nori sheets and spread the rice over them, leaving a small space at the top and bottom for sealing and making an indentation in the middle with a chopstick. Place some carrot, cucumber and spring onion in the middle with your umeboshi paste and roll up, sealing the end with a little water. Slice up each roll into 3 or 4cm slices and upend. Serve with soy sauce.

CHAPTER 2

Vegetables – In a league of their own when it comes to providing essential nutrients

The fact that vegetables, like fruits, are necessary for good health is hardly ground-breaking news... from a young age it's instilled into us to eat our greens and munch on carrots to help us see in the dark!

And with good reason, vegetables are an excellent source of fibre – the most fibrous of all are mustard and cress. They are also packed full of essential vitamins, minerals and cancer-fighting antioxidants.

In particular, cruciferous vegetables such as Brussels sprouts, cabbage, cauliflower and broccoli help kick-start your body's detoxifying enzymes that eliminate toxins from your system.

Are you getting your 5 a day?

Eating a variety of five fruit and vegetables a day could reduce deaths from heart disease, stroke and cancer by up to 20 per cent, according to the NHS Plan, a Department of Health document published back in 2000.

Not only that, fruit and veg can stop you piling on the pounds. They're low in fat and, as already mentioned, are packed with fibre. And because fibre fills you up, you're less likely to succumb to unhealthy calorie-laden snacks.

The bad news is that most of us aren't getting enough. According to the National Diet and Nutrition Survey, only 13 per cent of men and 15 per cent of women regularly achieve five a day with average intake below three.

Healthy eating tips – your way to 5 a day

- It can sometimes be difficult to squeeze in all five portions. But fresh, frozen, chilled, canned, 100 per cent juice and smoothies all count, as do dried fruit and veg. Although, bear in mind that potatoes don't count at all. Plus pasta sauces and fresh and tinned soups also contribute to your five a day – but check the nutritional information on the labels as you don't want to undo the goodness with lots of sugar, fat or salt. Around 80g of fruit and veg in a product counts as a portion.
- A portion of vegetables is three heaped tablespoons of carrots, peas or sweetcorn, or a cereal bowl of mixed salad. Three heaped tablespoons of beans and pulses such as lentils and chickpeas (for more examples, see the 'Seeds, beans and pulses – a good source of protein, fibre, vitamins and minerals' chapter on page 103) also count as a portion, but only count them once a day, even if you eat all three. That's because pulses don't contain as many nutrients.
- A portion of fruit is one medium apple or banana, two small satsumas or three dried apricots. You can only count a glass of 100 per cent fruit juice once a day, however many flavours you drink. Fibre is removed in processing so it's not as nutritious as a piece of fruit. A portion of dried fruit is one tablespoon but stick to one a day as it is high in sugar.
- Try something new every week. There are bound to be tons of fruit and veg varieties that you've never tasted – so vary what you buy and eat, rather than get into a rut of buying the same five things every time you go to the greengrocers. Aim for as many colours and textures as possible and five different choices every day. For example, five bananas would still only count as one portion.

A simple way to keep your mind sharp as you age

New research is constantly revealing more reasons why we should be upping our intake of vegetables. For example, US researchers from the Rush University Medical Center in Chicago have found that eating two or more servings of vegetables a day can help slow the age-related decline in cognitive function by up to 40 per cent, compared with a person who consumes few vegetables (*Neurology, 24 October 2006*).

In a six-year study funded by the National Institute on Aging, Dr Martha Clare Morris, of the Rush Institute for Healthy Aging, and colleagues, evaluated food frequency questionnaires completed by 3,718 Chicago residents aged 65 and older. Participants completed at least two of three cognitive function tests conducted at the beginning of the study and then after three and six years.

The researchers discovered that vegetable, but not fruit, consumption was associated with a reduced rate of cognitive decline. Of the different types of vegetables consumed by participants, green leafy vegetables had the strongest association to slowing the rate of cognitive decline. The study also found the older the person, the greater the slowdown in the rate of cognitive decline if that person consumed more than two servings of vegetables a day.

Commenting on the findings, Dr Morris said: "Compared to people who consumed less than one serving of vegetables a day, people who ate at least 2.8 servings of vegetables a day saw their rate of cognitive change slow by roughly 40 per cent. This decrease is equivalent to about five years of younger age."

Dr Morris added that the lack of benefit found for fruit was unanticipated. "It may be due to vegetables containing high amounts of vitamin E, which helps lower the risk of cognitive decline," she explained. "Vegetables, but not fruits, are also typically consumed with added fats such as salad dressings, and fats increase the absorption of vitamin E. Still, further study is required to understand why fruit is not associated with cognitive change."

While variety, as well as colour as detailed on page 7, is the key to making sure you're getting the maximum health benefits from vegetables in your diet, the following deserve a special mention for the remarkable therapeutic properties they possess.

It's also important to point out that the way you cook your veggies is very important in order to unlock their full goodness. Make sure you steam your vegetables rather than boil them, otherwise you risk losing many of the important nutrients they contain. If you do boil vegetables, the cooking water should be used for another culinary purpose, since boiling causes the leaching of the minerals they contain into the cooking water. For example, use the water for soup making. Stir frying is OK as long as you do not cook over a very high temperature and only cook the vegetables for a few minutes.

Ashitaba – News about this 'super food' from Japan is quickly spreading... make sure you don't miss out on its many benefits

A food that has been found to possess many medicinal properties, despite remaining relatively unheard of in the West, is the green leafy vegetable ashitaba (*Angelica Keiskei Koidzmi*). Indigenous to China and the Japanese islands of Izu, ashitaba has been an important part of the local diet for hundreds of years – used as a vegetable accompaniment at mealtimes and also drunk as a tea.

Ashitaba is a celery-like plant belonging to the Angelica family. Because it grows very fast, in the Japanese language it literally means 'leaves of tomorrow'. Now, mounting evidence suggests it may well prove to be an essential healing agent of tomorrow and indeed in the longer-term too.

Studies have shown that ashitaba can help improve overall health as well as help treat a number of medical complaints. These include weakened immunity, bacterial or viral infections, high blood pressure, high cholesterol, joint or muscular pain, and Type 1 and Type 2 diabetes. It also promotes detoxification of the blood, liver and kidneys.

Why ashitaba is an ideal food for vegans and vegetarians

It is not difficult to ascertain why ashitaba exerts so many positive effects on health when you consider the broad range of nutrients it contains – including 11 different types of vitamins and 13 minerals.

Nutritional analysis reveals that 100 grams of ashitaba contains the beta-carotene content equivalent to four carrots, the vitamin B2 content equivalent to 28 cloves of garlic, the vitamin C content equivalent to four lemons, and nine times the amount of iron found in spinach. It also contains vitamins B1, B3, B5, B6, biotin, folic acid, and the minerals calcium, magnesium, potassium, phosphorous, zinc, copper, manganese, sulphur and silicon.

Most plants are devoid of vitamin B12, which is normally only obtainable through meat, fish and eggs. However, ashitaba is a good source of this nutrient, making it an ideal supplement for strict vegetarians and vegans, who omit these foods from their diets and are at risk of suffering from a deficiency. A shortage of B12 can cause serious cognitive and nervous system problems, in addition to increasing the risk of cardiovascular disease and pernicious anaemia.

The list of therapeutic compounds in ashitaba is endless

Many researchers believe that ashitaba is effective against so many different medical problems as a result of its synergistic action – a combined effect of its various active components working together. In addition to the vitamin and minerals it contains, ashitaba also possesses lesser-known nutrients that also have specific health-related benefits. These include:

- **Chlorophyll.** Ashitaba is rich in chlorophyll, the green pigment present in plants that is responsible for collecting and storing energy from the sun. Because the chlorophyll molecule is almost identical to the haemoglobin molecule in red blood cells it is often referred to as 'nature's blood'. And one of its many attributes includes its ability to stimulate the production of red blood cells, which carry oxygen to the body's tissues. It is also an excellent agent for cleansing the blood and liver, and promotes the growth of 'friendly' intestinal bacteria.
- **Germanium.** This trace mineral has been found to promote the production of interferon, a substance produced in the body that works to prevent viruses and bacteria from penetrating the body's cells.
- **Coumarins.** These are potent antioxidants, which have been found to contain anti-carcinogenic properties (*Carcinogenesis 1997; 18: 1521-1527*). They are particularly abundant in ashitaba and other foods such as citrus fruit and celery.
- **Chalcones.** Unique to ashitaba is a class of flavonoid compounds called chalcones. Research has shown that they are potent antioxidants, protecting cells from free radical damage, which is associated with accelerating the ageing process and with many degenerative diseases, including cancer. They also suppress the excessive secretion of gastric juice in the stomach, which is often caused by stress and can lead to stomach ulcers. In addition they help strengthen the immune system, regulate blood pressure and cholesterol, and exhibit antiviral and antibacterial activities.

Chalcones have also been found to stimulate the production of Nerve Growth Factor (NGF), which is synthesised in minute amounts in the body and is essential in the development and survival of certain neurons (nerve cells) in the peripheral and central nervous system. NGF is believed to have the potential to alleviate Alzheimer's disease and peripheral neuropathy (a common neurological disorder resulting from damage to the peripheral nerves, which originate from the brain and spinal cord). In an animal study conducted by the Biomedical Group, in Takara, Japan, there was a 20 per cent increase in NGF concentration after taking ashitaba for just four days (*Ginny Bank and Rod Lenoble, Oxygen Radical Absorbance Capacity, Nutraceuticals World, September 2002*).

Helps disarm harmful free radicals and keeps blood sugar levels stable

Research published in the September 2002 issue of Nutraceuticals World, showed that ashitaba outperformed a range of herbs including sage, St. John's wort, camomile, dandelion, fennel, black tea and green tea for its antioxidant potential.

There is also mounting data to suggest that ashitaba has a regulating effect on blood sugar levels. In reviewing ashitaba, Dr Kevin Lance Jones, a licensed acupuncturist and orthomolecular medical doctor (OMD) from California, in the US, says: "There is a patient in Texas that has insulin-dependent (Type 1) diabetes that is currently taking the herb. He says that he now has to use less insulin because his blood sugar no longer spikes with attacks of hyperglycaemia. Another diabetes patient in Japan took ashitaba for six months and his blood sugar level dropped from 400 mg/dl to 150 mg/dl."

How to benefit from ashitaba

Eat raw or cooked. Stems can be lightly boiled and used like asparagus; leaves can be lightly boiled and eaten in place of spinach, or chopped and added to soups and stir-fries.

Eat your greens and your blood pressure will drop

Because vegetarians have lower rates of hypertension than meat eaters, it used to be thought that meat consumption causes high blood pressure. But tests have shown that eating meat, eggs or fat has little effect (*Nutrition Reviews 47(10): 291-300, 1989*).

The difference comes from the amount of green vegetables and fruit eaten, because of their high content of potassium, magnesium, vitamin C and fibre – which can lower blood pressure (*Lancet ii: 742-3, 1983*).

Magnesium is crucial for lowering blood pressure. A low magnesium intake correlated most closely with high blood pressure when the diets of 615 men were analysed (*Am. J. Clin. Nutr. 45(2): 469-75, 1987*). Aim to eat more magnesium-rich foods in your diet – in addition to green leafy vegetables, other good sources include nuts, seeds, dried peas and beans.

The vitamin C content in vegetables, like celery as mentioned earlier on page 4, is another powerful preventive – research shows that hypertension and strokes occur most frequently in people who eat the least vitamin C (*J. Hypertens. 12: 1071-75, 1990*).

How beetroot is making a comeback

Sweet, colourful and versatile, the humble beetroot has experienced something of a resurgence in popularity over the past few years. Chic restauranteurs are beginning to discover what home cooks have known all along: beetroot, whether roasted or boiled, pickled or puréed, adds a distinctive shot of colour to any meal.

Derived from the maritime sea beet, beetroot was highly esteemed as far back as the Roman times. Now, chefs are again making the most of its sweet, slightly nutty flavour and glorious red-purple colour.

The beetroot belongs to the same family as spinach and chard, the difference being that with beetroot both the leaves and root can be eaten. Beet greens (use in salads and stir frys) are higher in nutritional value than the roots as they are a richer source of calcium, iron and vitamins A & C. The roots are a very good source of folic acid, fibre, manganese and potassium, whereas both the greens and roots are rich in magnesium, phosphorous, iron and vitamin B6.

Usually when you buy fresh beetroot it will still have the leaves and stalks attached. To cook the beetroot, simply cut off the stalks but make sure you leave some of the stalk intact. By doing this it will help to stop the beetroot from losing its colour when you cook it and helps to hold in the nutrients.

The health benefits of beetroot are varied and include its stimulating effects on your liver's detoxification processes. It is one of the great cleansers and immune system strengtheners, having a beneficial effect on your entire system.

In addition, beetroot has for many years been used as a treatment for cancer throughout Europe. Specific anti-carcinogens are bound to its red colouring (a powerful pigment called betacyanin), which appear to be particularly effective against colon and stomach cancers. Beetroot also increases the uptake of oxygen by as much as 400 per cent.

Beetroot is good for your heart too as it contains soluble fibre which can help to reduce high blood cholesterol levels. It also contains the phytochemicals carotenoids and flavonoids, which help prevent LDL 'bad' cholesterol from being oxidised and deposited in the arteries.

Beetroot juice can help bring your blood pressure down

According to the results of a new UK study, drinking just 500ml of beetroot juice a day can significantly reduce blood pressure (*Hypertension – Journal of the American Heart Association, Published online ahead of print 4 February 2008, doi: 10.1161 / HYPERTENSIONAHA.107.103523*).

The benefits are linked to the nitrate content of the vegetable, and suggest an alternative explanation for the heart-healthy potential of vegetable-rich diets previously attributed to their antioxidant vitamin content.

Researcher Professor Amrita Ahluwalia of the William Harvey Research Institute at Barts and The London School of Medicine, said: "Our research suggests that drinking beetroot juice, or consuming other nitrate-rich vegetables, might be a simple way to maintain a healthy cardiovascular system, and might also be an additional approach that one could take in the modern day battle against rising blood pressure".

The researchers recruited 14 health volunteers and randomly assigned them to drink 500ml of beetroot juice or water during a 30 minute period. Blood pressure (BP) was measured every 15 minutes for one hour before and three hours after consuming the beverage, then every hour for six hours, with a final reading after 24 hours.

Commenting on the findings the researchers said that BP was 'substantially reduced' three hours after consuming the beetroot juice. Moreover, a degree of reduction continued to be observed until up to 24 hours after ingestion.

The decrease in BP correlated with peak increases in plasma nitrite concentration, they said, with the conversion of nitrate to nitrite occurring in the saliva by bacteria on the tongue. This nitrite-rich saliva was subsequently swallowed, and underwent further conversion in the acidic conditions of the stomach into nitric oxide or re-entered the circulation as nitrite.

"[The] reduction in BP correlated with the appearance and peak levels of nitrite in the circulation; an effect that was absent in individuals within whom the enterosalivary circuit was disrupted by avoidance of swallowing," said lead researcher Andrew Webb.

"These observations, together with the fact that plasma nitrite, and not nitrate, concentration correlated with the decreases in BP implicates nitrite as the likely functional mediator of the beetroot juice-induced effects on BP."

Commenting on the mechanism, the researchers stated that it was unknown how nitrite mediates blood pressure reductions, but noted that recent research has reported that nitrite can act as a potent vasodilator, which opens up blood vessels and improves circulation.

Beetroot soup – A delicious way to cleanse your system

This recipe serves 4 people

For this dish you will need the following ingredients:

500g beetroot, scrubbed and trimmed
3 tbsp extra virgin olive oil
1 large onion, halved and finely sliced
3 cloves of garlic, sliced
500ml vegetable stock
150g feta
2 tbsp snipped chives
Salt and freshly ground black pepper

To Prepare:

Heat the oil in a pan and add the onion and garlic. Allow to soften for approx. five minutes.

Grate the beetroot. Add to the softened onion, stir in a pinch of salt and pour in the stock and 500ml of cold water. Boil for 15 minutes, then cool for five. Add 50g of the feta and liquidize to a purée.

Sprinkle each serving with some more crumbled feta, the chives and a little freshly ground black pepper.

Broccoli provides you with an important defence against stomach ulcers and cancer

The fact that broccoli – an incredibly rich source of vitamins and minerals – is good for your health is nothing new. Its ability to boost immunity, detoxify your digestive system and liver, enhance mood, improve skin and fight cancer is well-documented.

But now scientists have discovered yet another reason to eat more of this healthful vegetable. Researchers at the Johns Hopkins School of Medicine in Baltimore and the French National Scientific Research Centre, recently discovered that a compound found in broccoli – sulforaphane – could help kill helicobacter pylori, or H pylori, the bacterium responsible for stomach ulcers and most stomach cancers.

Better still, the researchers found that the compound can even kill H pylori that has become resistant to antibiotics. Laboratory experiments showed that sulforaphane was able to kill the H pylori bacterium both inside and outside of cells. This is good news, as normally cells lining the stomach act as reservoirs for the bacteria – making it more difficult to eliminate.

Sulforaphane is also thought to help prevent cancer by boosting the production of phase 2 enzymes within cells, which detoxify carcinogens and free radicals. Although further trials are needed, preliminary findings have so far been extremely promising.

Research team leader and plant physiologist in the Department of Pharmacology and Molecular Sciences at the Johns Hopkins School of Medicine, Jed Fahey, stated: "In some parts of Central and South America, Africa and Asia, as much as 80 per cent to 90 per cent of the population is infected with helicobacter, likely linked to poverty and conditions of poor sanitation.

"If future clinical studies show that a food can relieve or prevent diseases associated with this bacterium in people, it could have significant public health implications in the United States and around the world... We've known for some time that sulforaphane had modest antibiotic activity. However, its potency against helicobacter, even those strains resistant to conventional antibiotics, was a pleasant surprise."

Spicy chicken and broccoli dish

This recipe serves 2 people

For this dish you will need the following ingredients:

75g wholewheat spaghetti
1 tsp extra virgin olive oil
2 skinless, boneless chicken breasts, cut into thin strips
200g broccoli, cut into florets
1 tbsp soy sauce
2 tbsp sweet chilli sauce
100g beansprouts
1 mild red chilli, deseeded and finely chopped
4 spring onions, thinly sliced
2 tsp sesame seeds, toasted

To prepare:

Cook the spaghetti in a pan of boiling water according to the packet instructions. Meanwhile, heat the oil in a wok and stir-fry the chicken for three minutes, then add the broccoli and chilli and stir-fry for a further two minutes.

Mix together the soy sauce, sweet chilli sauce and two tablespoons of water. Add to the pan and, once bubbling, stir in the beansprouts. Cook for a minute or so until the beansprouts look a little translucent.

Drain the spaghetti and add to the pan with the spring onions and sesame seeds. Stir together and serve piping hot.

The top 20 antioxidant vegetables

- Broccoli
- Celery
- Brussels sprouts
- Aubergine
- Spinach
- Kale
- Green beans
- Beetroot
- Cabbage
- Red pepper
- Carrots
- Cauliflower
- Garlic
- Lettuce (iceberg)
- Lettuce (leaf)
- Onion
- Potato
- Sweet potato
- Yellow squash
- Corn

Garlic – How to make sure you're taking full advantage of its heart-friendly properties

Root? Vegetable? Herb? Spice? Ask people what category garlic falls into and you'll probably hear each of those answers at least once – but only one is correct. Garlic is a vegetable, in the allium family along with leeks and onions.

But garlic has a unique characteristic. When you crush a garlic clove, a cascade of chemicals is released, activating the components of garlic that are believed to provide healthy benefits such as protection against bacterial and fungal infections, blood clots and high blood pressure.

Recent laboratory research at the University of Alabama in the US reveals the likely mechanism that makes garlic a heart helper. And according to a *HealthDay News* report, the UA team began their research just as you might begin making a pungent marinara sauce: They crushed the garlic.

The published study (*Proceedings of the National Academy of Sciences, "Hydrogen Sulfide Mediates the Vasoactivity of Garlic", Published online before print 19/10/07, www.pnas.org*) is a bit weighed down with highly technical chemistry jargon. So here's the layman's version:

After exposing human red blood cells to crushed garlic, the UA tests showed that the cells converted garlic-derived components called organic polysulphides into hydrogen sulphide, a molecule that protects blood vessels by reducing inflammation and relaxing vessel walls.

It's all in the preparation

So… if hydrogen sulphide helps keep blood vessels elastic and healthy, and garlic works with the body to create hydrogen sulphide, why are some garlic studies inconclusive or show little benefit for the heart?

According to Dr David Kraus, the lead UA researcher, if garlic is not prepared properly its benefits are negligible or lost altogether. And the key, apparently, is in the crushing. Dr. Kraus told *HealthDay* that he and his team not only crushed the garlic used in their study, they allowed about 15 minutes for the resulting chemical cascade to fully take effect (*"Garlic May Ward Off Heart Woes" Ed Edelson, HealthDay News, 16/10/07, www.healthday.com*).

Dr. Kraus also noted that some garlic trials have tested the vegetable as an LDL-lowering agent. Such research is bound to fail, he says, because the trials are looking for garlic activity that he calls 'impossible'. Another nutrition researcher confirmed this, telling *HealthDay* that hydrogen sulphide has no effect on cholesterol.

Of course, the UA study only gives us an insight into the effects of properly prepared fresh garlic. But according to Simon Mills and Kerry Bone in their textbook on botanical medicine, *Principles and Practice of Phytotherapy*, when garlic is dried in powered form at low temperatures, the garlic enzyme allinase and the active compound alliin remain intact, converting to allicin in the digestive tract, which is the same chemical chain of events that follows the crushing of a garlic clove.

How odour-free garlic supplements can help keep your arteries unclogged

Despite the fact that garlic is known to provide protection against a wide range of serious conditions, including heart disease and cancer, many people are put off because they don't want their breath to smell or because they suffer digestive problems after eating it.

While taking garlic supplements is an option, the question has always remained as to whether they are able to confer the same benefits. The good news is that recent research findings are suggesting that garlic does not have to be eaten raw or fresh to be effective.

US researchers at Pennsylvania State University have found that aged garlic extract (AGE), an odourless and concentrated form of the bulb, reduced cholesterol levels in the male participants they tested. Every day the men took either nine capsules containing 800mg of AGE or placebo for five months. At the end of the study, the men taking AGE showed a 7 per cent reduction in their total cholesterol levels, while their LDL ('bad') cholesterol levels dropped by 10 per cent. The placebo group showed no change.

According to Dr Yeh, a professor of Nutritional Biochemistry of Penn State's Department of Nutritional Sciences: "Aged garlic extract can be useful for the general public to help achieve the desired cholesterol level of 200 or less."

In another US study currently under review for publication, UCLA researchers conducted a double-blind randomised trial on 19 participants who consumed aged garlic extract or a placebo for one year. All of the participants underwent a test called electron beam tomography (EBT) to determine their atherosclerotic plaque levels at the study's onset and again after 12 months. While the placebo group experienced an average progression in plaque build-up of 22.2 per cent, progression in the group taking garlic was just 7.5 per cent. Blood tests also revealed improvements in high-density lipoprotein (HDL) cholesterol and homocysteine status in the group taking garlic. These results are extremely encouraging in the on-going fight against atherosclerosis and heart disease.

The recommended dosage for aged garlic extract is 1,000mg tablet taken one to two times a day.

Steamed garlic and lemon grass sea bass

This recipe serves 4 people

For this dish you will need the following ingredients:

1 ½ stems of lemon grass (finely sliced)
3 cloves of garlic (crushed or finely sliced)
4 x 175g sea bass fillets
200g runner beans (trimmed)
200g asparagus (trimmed)
Salt and pepper
Lemon olive oil (to make this add slices of lemon to a bottle of olive oil and leave for 24 hours to infuse)

To prepare:

Mix together the garlic and lemon grass and coat the sea bass fillets with it. Put the sea bass, asparagus and runner beans in a steamer and season with salt and pepper. Cook for six to eight minutes, until the fish is firm and white. Divide the seas bass and vegetables between four plates and drizzle with the lemon olive oil. Serve immediately. This dish goes well with cooked new potatoes.

Mushrooms possess a wide range of therapeutic actions

Mushrooms are a valuable health food – low in calories, high in vegetable proteins, chitin, iron, zinc, fibre, essential amino acids, vitamins and minerals. In particular, most mushrooms provide good amounts of vitamin C and the B vitamins, as well as the mineral calcium. They are also a good source of niacin, pantothenate and copper.

Three species of mushroom in particular have demonstrated phenomenal healing potential: maitake, shiitake and reishi.

These medicinal mushrooms have been shown to boost heart health, lower the risk of cancer, promote immune function, ward off viruses, bacteria, and fungus, reduce inflammation, combat allergies, help balance blood sugar levels, and support the body's detoxification mechanisms.

Recent studies have shown shiitake and reishi mushrooms are potential cancer-fighters. Shiitake mushrooms contain a compound called lentinan, which is being used as a cancer treatment in Japan. For more details on the cancer-fighting properties linked to reishi see the box below. And for a delicious yet simple to prepare dish that includes mushrooms, see the risotto recipe on page 74 or the asparagus and sautéed mushroom-filled omelette recipe on page 182.

How the reishi mushroom is proving vital in the fight against prostate cancer

According to Israeli scientists from the University of Haifa, the fungus *Ganoderma lucidum* – commonly known as the reishi mushroom – is able to suppress mechanisms involved in prostate cancer progression. These findings are extremely important, as every year nearly 35,000 cases of prostate cancer are diagnosed in the UK alone. The disease also causes 10,000 deaths in the UK each year.

Research concerning the possible anti-cancer benefits of various fungi conducted over the past few decades has mainly focused on their incredible immune-boosting abilities. As lead researcher Dr Ben-Zion Zaidman explained: "We already knew the mushroom could impede the development of cancer by affecting the immune

---

system. The in vitro trials we have done show that it attacks the cancer cells directly."

In the current study, Dr Zaidman, acting under the direction of Professors Eviatar Nevo and Solomon Wasser, from the University of Haifa's Institute of Evolution, and Dr Jamal Mahajna, from the Migal Galilee Technology Center, evaluated the ability of extracts from 68 different fungi to act from within the cell to interfere with the androgen (male hormone) receptor and inhibit cancer growth. The compounds from the fungi were extracted with solvents such as ether, ethyl acetate or ethanol that select molecules small enough to act from within the cells.

Out of 201 extracts, Dr Zaidman's research revealed 11 that interfered with androgen receptor activity (which controls prostate cancer growth) by more than 40 per cent, and among the 169 extracts evaluated for cancer cell growth inhibition, 14 were discovered to be active. Of these active compounds, extracts derived from the reishi mushroom exerted the greatest interference on androgen receptor function and cancer cell development.

Commenting on the findings, Dr Zaidman said: "Potential possibilities exist to establish research and development of bioactive metabolites from *Ganoderma lucidum* that could yield an anti-prostate cancer drug."

Mixed oriental mushroom risotto

This recipe serves 6 people

For this dish you will need the following ingredients:

225g (8oz) mixed oriental mushrooms
1 small onion, finely chopped
1 tbsp extra virgin olive oil

225g (8oz) risotto rice
150ml (¼pt) white wine
600ml (1pt) hot vegetable stock
Salt and freshly ground black pepper
50g (2oz) butter
2 crushed garlic cloves
30ml (2tbsp) fresh chopped parsley
Parmesan cheese, grated

To prepare:

Fry one small finely chopped onion in olive oil until softened. Add the risotto rice to the pan and stir continuously for one min.

Next, add the white wine and cook rapidly until nearly evaporated. Gradually add the hot vegetable stock, one ladle full at a time. Simmer gently, allowing the stock to be absorbed before adding the next ladle full. Continue, stirring frequently until the rice is tender (see the packet instructions for cooking times). Season with salt and freshly ground black pepper.

Meanwhile, in a separate frying pan, melt the butter and add the garlic cloves. Fry for one to two minutes then add the mixed oriental mushrooms and cook until tender and browned (add firmest ones such as shiitake first, delicate oyster and enoki last).

Season well, add the fresh chopped parsley and gently mix into the risotto, pouring over any remaining garlic butter. Grate the parmesan cheese on top and serve.

Onions can protect your bones and help prevent osteoporosis

Like garlic, onions have also been found to lower high blood pressure, reduce cholesterol levels and protect against heart disease. Research has revealed that they are also able to reduce the risk of diabetes, attack bacteria that cause infection and reduce the risk of certain cancers. With regards to the latter, scientists have identified a compound in onions called quercetin, which is a powerful antioxidant and cancer-attacking agent.

But its benefits don't end there. In an animal study, researchers at the University of Bern in Switzerland found a compound in white onions – a peptide called GPCS – that appears to prevent bone loss and osteoporosis.

These findings are promising, as osteoporosis – a disease described by the World Health Organization as the leading global healthcare problem after heart disease – currently affects 30 million people (predominantly women) worldwide.

The researchers found that treating bone cells that had been exposed to parathyroid hormone (which stimulates bone loss) with GPCS significantly inhibited the loss of bone minerals, including calcium, when compared to cells that were not exposed to GPCS (*Journal of Agricultural and Food Chemistry, 4 May 2005*).

Further studies are now needed to determine whether these same benefits apply to human bone health.

In the meantime, eating plenty of onions may offer a good precaution against bone loss and is also an excellent way of maintaining overall good health – especially as onions have other known health benefits, such as inhibiting the growth of liver and colon cancer cells.

Go continental with a delicious French onion tart

This recipe serves 4 people

For this dish you will need the following ingredients:

3 tbsp extra virgin olive oil
2 tbsp brown sugar
1 tbsp balsamic vinegar
2 tbsp wholegrain mustard
2 garlic gloves, crushed
6 onions, finely sliced
50g Gruyere cheese, grated
Salt and pepper
Shortcut pastry

To prepare:

Heat the olive oil in a non-stick pan and add your finely sliced onions. Cover and cook gently for about 15 minutes, stirring occasionally, until they become soft. Keep a close eye on them to ensure they don't burn.

Add the crushed garlic, sugar and vinegar and cook for a further five minutes, or until the onions are caramelised. Salt and pepper to taste.

Preheat your oven to 200C or Gas Mark 5. If you want a big 26cm tart, roll your pastry and put it in your tart dish. Do some cuts with a fork all over, cover the pastry with dried beans to cook the pastry without the filling. Bake the pastry for 10 minutes.

After 10 minutes, take out the now cooked tart, empty any beans and spread inside the pastry a spoon of wholegrain mustard. Pour in the onion mixture and cover slightly with Gruyere cheese. Return to bake for 10 minutes.

Don't overlook the merits of the humble potato... especially the sweet variety

With so much media focus on low-carbohydrate diets lately, one carb in particular has received an undeservedly bad rap – the humble potato.

Unlike refined carbohydrates, like white bread and biscuits, which provide little nutritional value, potatoes supply a number of important vitamins and minerals. For example, they contain approximately 40 per cent more potassium – essential for the proper functioning of your muscles and nerves – than bananas. They're also a rich source of iron, which helps your body convert food to energy and makes it better able to withstand infection.

Potatoes also provide vitamin C, which is essential for maintaining healthy connective tissue and healing wounds, and B vitamins, which help your body make healthy red blood cells and amino acids. The skins are also an excellent source of fibre.

In addition to these nutritional benefits, potatoes are also credited with having further health advantages. For example, a traditional remedy for mild skin burns is to apply a slice of raw potato to the affected area. This cools the skin down and reduces the flow of blood to the site of the burn – preventing pain, swelling and blistering.

Researchers have also discovered that potatoes contain high levels of antioxidants – natural chemicals which help fight harmful free radicals that are linked to accelerating the ageing process and increasing the risk of serious diseases like cancer, heart disease, stroke and diabetes.

When free radicals damage your cells, they release another toxic compound called Malondialdehyde (MDA) – high concentrations of which are an indicator that extensive damage has already been waged on the body by free radicals. Promising research findings from scientists working at the Department of Functional Biology, Faculty of Medicine, University of Oviedo, in Spain, have revealed that potatoes can help prevent a build up of MDA by up to 18 per cent (*J Am Diet Assoc. 2003103(11): 1480-7*).

However, the way you cook potatoes is important. Avoid fried potatoes at all costs as the frying process has been found to increase the concentration of a harmful toxin called acrylamide, which is implicated in causing cancer. Opt for baked potatoes instead, as leaving the skin on helps retain their nutritional value.

Better still, opt for sweet potatoes, which are a veritable treasure trove of vitamins and minerals. They are a first-rate provider of vitamin A and beta-carotene (a compound your body converts into vitamin A), both of which promote healthy skin, hair and eyesight. In fact, a serving of sweet potatoes has four times the recommended daily allowance for beta-carotene. Believe it or not, one cup of cooked sweet potato provides so much beta-carotene that it would take 23 cups of broccoli to provide the same amount!

Sweet potatoes also contain significant amounts of vitamins C and are a fair source of vitamin E. Along with beta-carotene, these vitamins make up the terrific trio of antioxidant nutrients scientists believe may help prevent heart disease and cancer, bolster the immune system, and even slow the ageing process. One medium sweet potato provides nearly half of your daily requirement of vitamin C. As if all this weren't good enough, sweet potatoes are also a great source of dietary fibre – when eaten with the skin, they offer more fibre than oatmeal!

Vegetarian shepherd's pie with sweet potato

This recipe serves 4 people

For this dish you will need the following ingredients:

4 large sweet potatoes (peeled and chopped)
Nutmeg (pinch of)
2 tbsp extra virgin olive oil
2 onions (chopped)
2 celery sticks (chopped)
3 carrots (chopped)
2 courgettes (chopped)
400g can chopped tomatoes
2 tbsp of tomato purée
100g red lentils
3 tbsp pesto
425ml vegetable stock

To prepare:

Preheat your oven to 180C/350F/Gas Mark 4

Fry the onion in the extra virgin olive oil for 10 minutes. Add the celery, courgettes, and carrots and fry for five minutes. Stir in the stock, tomatoes, tomato purée and lentils. Bring to the boil and then cover and simmer for 20 minutes, until the lentils are tender. Season, stir in the pesto and tip into a large ovenproof dish.

Meanwhile, cook the potatoes in boiling water for approximately 15 minutes or until just tender.

Drain the potatoes and mash, adding the nutmeg. Spoon the mash over the lentil and vegetable mixture, sealing it in. Bake for approximately 20 minutes, or until the top is golden brown.

Good news for Type 1 diabetics: adding pumpkin to your diet could help regulate your blood sugar levels

Pumpkins are packed fill of beta-carotene – an antioxidant with properties that help improve immune function and reduce the risk of chronic diseases such as cancer and heart disease.

Pumpkins are also high in lutein and zeaxanthin, which scavenge free radicals in the lens of the eye and help prevent the formation of cataracts and reduce the risk of macular degeneration, a serious eye problem that usually results in blindness. Besides these nutrients, pumpkins also contain good levels of iron, zinc, calcium, vitamin C, potassium and fibre.

Plus pumpkin seeds are a great source of protein, essential fatty acids, copper, iron, magnesium, manganese, phosphorus, and zinc. They help promote good prostate health, lower high cholesterol, improve bladder function, alleviate depression, and have potent anti-inflammatory properties.

According to the results of a recent animal study, an extract from pumpkin (Cucurbita ficifolia) may improve blood glucose levels in diabetics, in addition to exerting a beneficial antioxidant effect (*Journal of the Science of Food and Agriculture, Volume 87, Issue 9, Pages 1753-1757*).

If the research, conducted by scientists from the East China Normal University, can be reproduced in humans, then the consumption of pumpkin extract could promote the regeneration of damaged pancreatic cells in diabetics and boost levels of insulin-producing beta cells and insulin in the blood.

According to researchers Tao Xia and Qin Wang: "The present

study provides substantial evidence to demonstrate the hypoglycaemic action of C. ficifolia fruit extract as well as its role as antioxidant agent and thus reveals a mechanism for its cytoprotective action."

Lead researcher, Tao Xia, added: "Pumpkin extract is potentially a very good product for pre-diabetic persons, as well as those who have already developed diabetes."

The rats used in this study modeled Type 1 diabetes, but the researchers believe the pumpkin extract may also play a beneficial role in Type 2 diabetes. Type 1 diabetes occurs when people are not able to produce any insulin after the cells in the pancreas have been damaged, which is thought to be an autoimmune response.

Tao Xia and Qin Wang divided 12 diabetic rats and 12 normal rats into two groups, one was fed a normal diet and the other fed the normal diet supplemented with the pumpkin extract for 30 days.

At the end of the study, the researchers found that diabetic rats fed the extract had only 5 per cent less plasma insulin and 8 per cent fewer insulin-positive (beta) cells compared to normal healthy rats.

The mechanism behind these potential benefits was proposed to be due to both antioxidants and D-chiro-inositol – a molecule that mediates insulin activity. Boosting insulin levels has the effect of lowering blood sugar levels, which reduces levels of oxidative oxygen species that damage beta cell membranes, preventing further damage and allowing for some regeneration.

However, the researchers were quick to point out that beta cell levels in the diabetic rats are unlikely ever to reach that of healthy controls, because some of the cells will have been damaged beyond repair.

The researchers concluded: "Thus our studies support the notion that supplementation of C. ficifolia fruit extract to diabetic patients would help in achieving good glycaemic and metabolic control and prevent long-term complications as a result of the protection offered by its antioxidant action; probably preserving the residual β-cell mass without further loss."

As well as making the delicious pumpkin soup below, take advantage of this vegetable's numerous health benefits by trying the pumpkin curry on page 141 too.

Hearty pumpkin, pepper and coriander soup

This dish serves 2 people

For this dish you will need the following ingredients:

1 small pumpkin
2 red peppers
2 tbsp olive oil
1 onion (chopped)
3 cloves garlic (crushed)
½ tsp juniper seeds
100g celery (chopped)
2 small red chillies (deseeded and finely chopped)
1 litre vegetable stock
2 tbsp crème fraiche
Large bunch of fresh coriander (chopped)
Salt and pepper
Pinch of paprika

To prepare:

Preheat the oven to 200C/400F/Gas Mark 6.

Quarter the pumpkin and remove the seeds (don't throw them away though as they make a delicious, healthy snack when roasted). Cut the red peppers in half, remove the seeds and place them with the pumpkin onto a roasting tray. Drizzle the flesh with a little olive oil and place in the pre-heated oven to roast for approximately 40 minutes.

Remove from the oven. Scrape the flesh from the skin of the pumpkin and put to one side along with the roasted pepper.

Heat a little olive oil in a saucepan; add the chopped onion, crushed garlic, juniper seeds, celery and red chillies. Cook for a few minutes until the onions and celery are soft. Add the pumpkin and red peppers, the stock and finally the chopped coriander. Bring to the boil, reduce the heat and allow to simmer for about 15 minutes.

Season with salt and pepper and then process the soup in a blender to make it smooth.

Serve with a spoonful of crème fraiche over the top sprinkled with a little paprika.

Spinach is packed with important, disease-fighting nutrients

We all know that Popeye made himself super strong by eating spinach, but you may be surprised to learn that he may also have been protecting himself against osteoporosis, heart disease, colon cancer, arthritis, high blood pressure, constipation and anaemia in the process.

Spinach is one of the most nutritious of the leafy green vegetables – it's packed full of calcium, folic acid, vitamin K, energy-promoting iron, vitamin C, fibre, carotenoids, lutein and bioflavonoids.

For optimal nutrition eat spinach raw – such as in sandwiches (in place of lettuce), or in salads. For a delicious spinach salad, toss baby spinach leaves with avocado, pistachio nuts and shaved parmesan cheese. You can always add some olives or sun-dried tomatoes for extra flavour.

The calcium content is responsible for its ability to strengthen bones and help ward off osteoporosis. The A and C vitamins in spinach plus the fibre, folic acid, magnesium and other nutrients help control cancer, especially colon, lung and breast cancers. Folate also lowers the blood levels of a substance called homocysteine – a protein that damages arteries and puts you at risk of heart disease. The flavonoids in spinach help protect against age-related memory loss.

Spinach's secret weapon, lutein, makes it one of the best foods to prevent cataracts, as well as age-related macular degeneration, the leading cause of preventable blindness in the elderly. Foods rich in lutein are also thought to help prevent cancer.

Please note: People with kidney or bladder stones should avoid spinach because its oxalic content can exacerbate stones.

Spinach, avocado and beetroot salad

This recipe serves 4 people

For this dish you will need the following ingredients:

250g spinach
1 bunch beetroot
2 tbsp walnut oil
1 small red onion, minced
1 tsp olive oil
splash red wine vinegar
1 avocado
Pepper and salt

To prepare:

Wash beetroot and cut off any leaves. Soak the leaves in a basin of cold water with the spinach. Steam the beetroot until they can be pierced easily with a skewer, then gently rub off the skins with your fingers.

Slice beetroot thickly and put into separate bowls. While the beetroot is still warm, sprinkle half the walnut oil into each bowl and add a little pepper.

Sauté onion in oil in a small pan for two minutes and divide between beetroot. Shake over red wine vinegar and taste for salt and sharpness.

Gently dry salad leaves and arrange on a flat platter. Peel and slice avocado and arrange amongst greens. Combine beetroots gently and quickly tumble over leaves with all the juices.

Researchers reveal how watercress plays a vital role in the prevention of cancer

Gram for gram, watercress contains as much vitamin C as oranges, more calcium than milk and more iron than spinach. It's a good source of folic acid, and is literally bursting with beta-carotene and vitamin A equivalents, which help promote healthy skin and eyes. It also contains antioxidants, which can help to mop up potentially harmful free radicals, and compounds known as glucosinolates which appear to have anti-cancer properties.

Researchers from the University of Ulster, in Northern Ireland, recently discovered that consuming watercress on a regular basis can prevent DNA damage – a key risk factor in the development of cancer (*American Journal of Clinical Nutrition, Feb 2007, Vol 85, No*

2, Pages 504-510). This is an important finding as over 150,000 people die from cancer every year in the UK, with one in three people predicted to develop the disease at some stage in their life.

The study involved 30 healthy men and 30 healthy women (average age of 33), half of whom were smokers. The participants were randomized to consume their usual diet or receive the addition of a bowlful (85 grams) of raw watercress each day for eight weeks.

After a seven week period, in which no watercress was consumed, the subjects switched regimens for a further eight weeks. Fasting blood samples were collected at the beginning and end of each eight week phase of the trial and several measures of lymphocyte DNA damage assessed. Plasma lutein, retinol, alpha-tocopherol and beta-carotene levels were also measured.

The researchers found that significant reductions in DNA damage occurred when the participants consumed watercress. These reductions were found to be greatest among those participants who were smokers.

In addition to reducing DNA damage in the white blood cells (lymphocytes), watercress consumption was also associated with a 9.4 per cent reduction in DNA damage to lymphocytes when challenged with free-radical (cancer-causing) toxins generating hydrogen peroxide. Better still, plasma lutein levels were found to double following the consumption of watercress, and beta-carotene concentrations rose by approximately one third.

The researchers believe that watercress may exert its protective effect on the genes due to its rich antioxidant content – in particular, lutein and beta-carotene. Analysis of watercress leaves detected several beneficial phenolic components such as rutin, as well as a number of glucosinolates, which may also contribute to its protective effect. The difference in beta-carotene levels between smokers and non-smokers in this study could be due to a greater requirement of the vitamin by individuals who smoke.

Commenting on the findings, lead researcher Professor Ian Rowland said: "Our findings are highly significant. Population studies have shown links between higher intakes of cruciferous vegetables like watercress, and a reduced risk of a number of cancers. However, such studies don't give direct information about causal effects. What makes this study unique is it involves people eating watercress in easily achievable amounts, to see what impact that might have on known bio-markers of cancer risk, such as DNA damage. Most studies to date have relied on tests conducted in test tubes or in animals, with chemicals derived from cruciferous vegetables.

"Blood cell DNA damage is an indicator of whole body cancer risk, and the results support the theory that consumption of watercress is linked to an overall reduced risk of cancer at various sites in the body."

Watercress and goat's cheese salad

This recipe serves 2 people

For this dish you will need the following ingredients:

1 x 85g bag watercress
1 red pepper
1 red onion, sliced
2 tbsp pine nuts
1 tbsp olive oil
1 (50g) goat's cheese, crumbled
2 tsp balsamic vinegar
salt and freshly ground black pepper

To prepare:

Preheat the oven to 200C/400F/Gas Mark 6.

Place the whole peppers on the middle shelf of the oven and roast for 20 minutes or until the skin has begun to brown. Toss the onions, pine nuts and olive oil together in a small baking tray and roast with the peppers for 10 minutes. Stir the vinegar and salt and pepper into the onions and set aside.

Carefully remove the peppers from the oven and transfer to a plastic bag, leave to cool – this helps 'sweat' the skin off the peppers. Peel away the pepper skin and remove the seeds. Slice the flesh into strips.

Empty the watercress into a salad bowl. Add the goat's cheese, sliced peppers, onions, pine nuts and any pan juices. Toss lightly to mix and serve.

CHAPTER 3

Grains – How to make sure you're eating the right kind

Grains in their pure form are an excellent source of fibre, vitamins and minerals. The problem that exists, particularly here in the West, is that the milling process has depleted many of these important nutrients from the grains we consume. The worst culprit is white, refined grain – such as white bread and white pasta – which is nutrient-free to a large extent and can cause blood sugar fluctuations, cravings and mood swings.

In addition, the chemicals added to flour, such as bleaching agents – helping white bread to appear even whiter for example – greatly lessens its nutritional value. In some cases, brown bread – which many people assume to be healthier than white – can simply be white bread coloured brown. Worse still, these bleaching agents are powerful oxidizing substances that increase the risk of free radical production that contribute to cell damage and toxicity; they also increase the risk of allergies developing.

Many health problems arising from eating wheat are normally associated with incomplete digestion of the gluten it contains. Coeliacs have a particularly adverse reaction to gluten, which can cause symptoms such as diarrhoea, weight loss, gas, abdominal pain, vomiting and weakness. Gluten is also present in rye, barley and oats.

But even eating too many wheat-based products like bread and pasta can cause a wheat allergy or intolerance to develop. A wheat intolerance has also been linked to triggering irritable bowel syndrome (IBS) symptoms in many sufferers.

Common foods that contain wheat are bread, pasta, cakes, biscuits, pastry and wheat-based breakfast cereals. It is also present as an ingredient in many sauces and ready meals.

The best choice is wholemeal bread for its rich fibre content, although it should be eaten in moderation to avoid an allergy developing. However, the best source of fibre is plant fibre. Not only can fibre enhance your weight-loss efforts by helping you feel full for longer as a result of slowing down the time it takes for your stomach to empty, but it also possesses numerous health-related benefits.

Fibre could help postmenopausal women lower their cholesterol... and lose inches from their hips and waist

Good news for postmenopausal women. US researchers have discovered an easy way for this population group to lose weight and maintain good health... simply by following a healthy diet and increasing their fibre intake (*Journal of Nutrition, August 2006*).

The study led by Dr Alok Bhargava at the University of Houston analyzed data from 994 women enrolled in the Women's Health Trial: Feasibility Study in Minority Populations. In this study, one group of women were given advice by a nutritionist over a one year period concerning reducing fat and increasing whole grains, fruits and vegetables; while a control group received pamphlets which provided information on healthy eating.

Dietary intake was determined via questionnaires administered at the beginning of the study and at six and 12 months. Height, weight, waist and hip circumferences were measured and blood samples were analysed for lipids, the hormone oestradiol, serum hormone binding globulin (SHBG – reduced levels of which have been associated with an increased risk of diabetes), glucose, and insulin before beginning the study and at its conclusion.

At the end of the 12 months, women who received the nutritional advice experienced a greater decrease in LDL ('bad') cholesterol levels, and a greater increase in SHBG compared to the control group.

These changes coincided with a reduction in saturated fat and calories, and an increase in dietary fibre. Women in the treatment group also experienced a reduction in weight and hip and waist circumference. Analysis of the data revealed greater fibre intake associated with lower insulin and triglycerides, and higher HDL (the 'good' form of cholesterol) levels in this group.

Commenting on the findings, Dr Bhargava, said: "The results from our comprehensive analysis of the WHTFSMP data demonstrated the importance of reducing central obesity in particular and increasing the intakes of dietary fibre for improving the lipid, lipoprotein, and hormonal profiles of postmenopausal women."

A European Investigation into Cancer (EPIC) study, revealed how individuals who consumed the highest amounts of fibre in their diets almost halved their risk of developing colon cancer, compared to those who only ate moderate amounts. It has also been found to help lower elevated cholesterol levels, control blood sugar levels and keep you regular.

Now, there's even more good news linked to eating a high-fibre diet, as researchers have established an association between fibre consumption and reduced levels of C-reactive protein (CRP) – a marker of inflammation. In particular, elevated CRP levels have been strongly implicated in increasing the risk of inflammation that causes cardiovascular disease.

Researchers came to this conclusion after analysing information gathered from the 1999 to 2000 National Health and Nutrition Examination Survey (NHANES), which included CRP level measurements of 4,900 adults. The intake of various nutrients was also calculated from reports provided by the study participants regarding what foods they consumed. Data on the daily consumption of fibre, total fat, saturated fatty acids, monounsaturated fatty acids, polyunsaturated fatty acids, protein, carbohydrates, total calories and cholesterol was provided. The researchers also took into account demographic variables such as age and gender, and cardiovascular risk factors such as smoking and alcohol consumption.

When fibre intake was assessed, participants whose consumption of fibre was in the top 50 per cent had a significantly lower risk of elevated CRP than the remaining half, with those in the top one-fourth having a 23 per cent lower CRP level on average than individuals in the lowest quarter of fibre intake. Not only was fibre found to reduce CRP levels but a high saturated fat intake was found to raise them.

So, to prevent heart disease eat more fibre-rich foods – fruit and vegetables are good sources and will also have the added health benefit of providing you with essential vitamins, minerals and antioxidants. Other foods to include more of in your diet for their high fibre content are legumes, kidney and pinto beans, oats, seeds, nuts, brown rice and whole grain cereals.

Not only that, but by eating more fibre and magnesium-rich grains you may be able to lower your risk of developing diabetes by as much as 27 per cent, according to the findings of a German study (*Archives of Internal Medicine 2007, Volume 167, Pages 956-965*).

This finding is extremely important as the UK is facing a huge increase in the number of cases of diabetes. According to the charity Diabetes UK, the number of people diagnosed with this disease, which currently stands at around 1.8 million, could reach 3 million by 2010. One of the main reasons behind this increase is our sedentary lifestyles coupled with our growing reliance on processed and sugar-rich foods.

Researchers from the German Institute of Human Nutrition Potsdam-Rehbruecke, used a prospective study of about 25,000 subjects (9,702 men and 15,365 women) with an average age of 49.6 years. The study population was part of the European Prospective Investigation into Cancer and Nutrition (EPIC)-Potsdam. Diets were assessed using a semi-quantitative 148-item food frequency questionnaire (FFQ) and studied for an average of seven years, during which time 844 cases of Type 2 diabetes were diagnosed.

Lead researcher Matthias Schulze and his co-workers calculated that the consumption of fibre through cereal, bread and other grain products (cereal fibre) was associated with a reduced risk of diabetes. Those with the highest fibre intake (an average of 29 grams per day) were calculated to have a 27 per cent lower risk than those with the lowest intake (an average of 15.1 grams per day). No difference in the reduction of risks was observed between soluble or insoluble fibre.

The researchers also conducted a meta-analysis of nine studies of fibre and eight studies of magnesium intake. After pooling the data, the researchers found that the highest consumption of cereal fibre was associated with a 33 per cent reduction in the risk of diabetes, while those who consumed the most magnesium had a 23 per cent lower risk, compared to those who consumed the least.

Low magnesium levels (hypomagnesemia) have been linked to lower activity of insulin receptors, reducing the effectiveness of insulin and leading to insulin resistance.

Commenting on the findings Matthias Schulze, said: "The evidence from our study and previous studies, summarized by means of meta-analysis, strongly supports that higher cereal fibre and magnesium intake may decrease diabetes risk. Whole grain foods are therefore important in diabetes prevention."

The difference between soluble and insoluble fibre

Soluble fibre slows the digestion of food, giving the body time to absorb nutrients. It prolongs the time food stays in the stomach, helping sugar to be released and absorbed more slowly into your system. Most doctors believe that eating foods rich in soluble fibre helps prevent symptoms of irritable bowel syndrome and relieve them if they do occur.

Soluble fibre foods are those more commonly thought of as starches, like oatmeal, barley, rice cereals, corn meal and potatoes. But soluble fibre is also found in carrots, yams, sweet potatoes, turnips, beets, squash, pumpkins, mushrooms, chestnuts, avocados, bananas, oranges, applesauce and mangos.

Insoluble fibre passes through your body largely intact, increasing the speed at which food moves through the stomach and intestines. Most of the foods people think of as high in fibre, such as wholewheat, bran products, and raw, leafy green vegetables, are actually high in insoluble fibre.

Unlike soluble fibre, foods containing insoluble fibre seem to increase irritation in those with gastrointestinal problems. In addition, you should be aware that wheat (and other cereal) bran contains compounds called phytates that actually block the absorption of minerals (mainly iron, zinc and calcium) in the gut. So eating lots of All Bran or adding spoonfuls of wheat bran to your food in the belief that it is doing you good, can sometimes lead to deficiency problems.

Oats are also good to include in your diet, not only because they are rich in fibre but because they are high in phosphorous too, which is beneficial for the brain and nervous system. Having a bowl of porridge each morning provides you with energy throughout the day and also helps prevent high cholesterol. Or, as an alternative, start your day with a refreshing fruit and oat smoothie – see the recipe on page 100 for more details.

Buckwheat – although technically a fruit rather than a grain – is rich in omega-3 fatty acids, B vitamins, minerals and essential amino acids. Further health benefits linked to buckwheat were uncovered by Spanish researchers who wanted to find out if buckwheat might also act as a prebiotic – a non-digestible carbohydrate that prompts the growth of 'friendly' bacteria (probiotics) in the digestive tract that help limit the numbers of harmful bacteria, aid digestion, and support immune function.

For 30 days the scientists fed 10 laboratory rats a diet that included buckwheat. An additional group of 10 rats were fed the same diet, but without buckwheat. At the end of the trial, the intestines of the rats were analysed and compared. Researchers found that the rats receiving buckwheat had a significantly greater amount of friendly bacteria than those of the control group, as well as three types of beneficial bacteria that were not present in the controls (*Nutrition Research, Volume 23, Issue 6, June 2003, pp 803-814*).

Quinoa is a good alternative to wheat too. It is an excellent source of amino acids, calcium and iron. See the tasty quinoa and tofu loaf recipe on page 98 for a delicious way to benefit from it.

Opt for brown rice rather than white as it is rich in vitamins, minerals, proteins and lipids that help maintain good health.

Savoury brown rice nutty salad

This recipe serves 4 people

For this dish you will need the following ingredients:

720g brown rice
240g spring onions, chopped
90g canned sweet corn
60g cashew nuts
60g raisins
1½ tbsp soy sauce
3 tbsp extra virgin olive oil
80g red pepper, chopped

To prepare:

Cook the rice according to the instructions on the packet.

Then, simply mix all the other ingredients with the cooked rice in a large bowl and enjoy.

Quinoa and tofu loaf

This dish serves 3-4 people

For this dish you will need the following ingredients:

100g of quinoa grain
100g of tofu
100g of rice flour
1 tsp of bicarbonate of soda
½ tsp of cream of tartar
¼ tsp of tartaric acid
Salt

¼ pint of water or milk
1 tsp of sugar
25g of fat or cooking oil

To prepare:

Soak the quinoa grain in boiling water for 10 minutes and then drain. Leave the grain to soak in one pint of water overnight and drain before using. Liquidise the soaked quinoa with the tofu to a smooth purée in a blender and beat in the milk. Mix all the dry ingredients for the bread together with one tablespoon of oil. Fold the flour mixture into the purée. Place the mixture 1inch deep into a shallow 10inch square baking tray lined with non-stick paper. Bake in a preheated oven 220C (Gas Mark 7) for 35-45 minutes. Check to see that the bread is cooked using a skewer through the middle (if the skewer comes out clean then this means the bread is cooked). A part-cooked loaf can be turned over on the baking tray to help ensure even cooking.

Spiced prawn, avocado and bulgar wheat salad with salmon pancake rolls

This recipe serves 4 people

For this dish you will need the following ingredients:

75g bulgar wheat
300g jumbo king prawns
2 tbsp chilli dipping sauce
5 tbsp of extra virgin olive oil
6 tbsp fresh orange juice
2 large avocados
8 radishes thinly sliced
100g frozen soybeans, defrosted (known as edamame in Japan)
10g coriander leaves, chopped

10g parsley leaves, chopped
4 ready-made pancakes
200g smoked salmon, thinly sliced
10cm piece cucumber thinly sliced
Salt and freshly ground black pepper

To prepare:

Put the bulgar wheat in a serving bowl and pour over enough boiling water to just cover. Leave to soak for 15 minutes.

Meanwhile, soak the prawns in the chilli dipping sauce. Whisk the olive oil into the orange juice and submerge the sliced avocado in the mixture.

Take a fork and fluff up the grains of bulgar wheat to separate them. Mix in the radish, soybeans and herbs, and season to taste.

Add the avocado and dressing to the prawns and chilli sauce, and gently mix.

For the salmon rolls, lay the pancakes flat and divide the salmon between them, leaving 3cm clear at the side furthest away. Do the same with the cucumber and season with pepper. Roll up loosely, so they don't split. Put in the fridge until ready to serve with the salad. You may prefer to serve the pancake cut in half with the ends cut off.

Kick-start your day with a refreshing fruit and oat smoothie

This drink serves 1-2 people

For this drink you will need the following ingredients:

Handful of ripe strawberries

1 banana, peeled and sliced
25g porridge oats
1 tbsp honey
150ml natural yoghurt
100ml apple juice

To prepare:

Place all the ingredients in a blender or food processor and blend to
a smooth, thick drink.

CHAPTER 4

Seeds, beans and pulses – A good source of protein, fibre, vitamins and minerals

Beans have many health benefits linked to them. Flaxseed and soyabeans in particular have both been shown to help prevent a number of diseases. Scientists at the Beltsville Human Nutrition Research Center in Maryland in the US, designed a study to test the beneficial effects of these two nutrients on liver steatosis (excess liver fat accumulation – a pre-diabetic condition) and hypertriglyceridemia (elevated triglyceride levels – a prominent marker for heart disease).

Two groups of rats were used in the study: one group was lean, while the other was a 'SHR/N-cp' rat – a variety considered to be a genetic model of obesity. Each of the two groups were then separated into sub-groups which were fed diets that delivered 20 per cent of energy through either a flaxseed meal, soy protein, or (for a control group) a milk-based protein called casein.

After six months, analysis of the livers and plasma showed that while the obese rats experienced far more fat build-up in the liver than the lean rats, those of both groups that were fed flaxseed showed far less liver fat accumulation. Additionally, triglyceride blood levels were lowered by almost 40 per cent in lean rats fed flaxseed, and more than one-third in the obese rats that received flaxseed.

Overall, both the lean and obese rats fed flaxseed experienced a significantly greater drop in triglycerides and reduced liver fat accumulation than those fed soy protein. (Rats fed soy and flax far outperformed those fed casein in all categories) (*Journal of the American College of Nutrition, Vol. 22, No. 2, 157-164, 2003*).

The results of the Beltsville test were not entirely a surprise, as flaxseed contains lignans, a good source of alpha-linolenic acid, which is converted by the body into omega-3 fatty acids. This helps improve cell function in the lining of the heart and blood vessels, lowers triglyceride levels, and inhibits platelet clumping.

Soy – Boosting your intake could reduce your risk of cancer

Soy is one of nature's most magnificent foods and it has a diverse range of health benefits – from regulating blood sugar levels and combating constipation to alleviating the symptoms of premenstrual syndrome and the menopause.

Soya beans are the most nutritious of all beans. High in fibre, they are also an excellent source of non-animal protein – able to lower high blood pressure and cholesterol levels. They have also been shown to reduce the risk of heart disease.

One of the areas where soy is proving particularly beneficial is in the fight against cancer. Research has shown that chemicals present in soy, known as isoflavones, can help lower the risk of breast, prostate, colon, ovarian and cervical cancers.

Now there is further evidence of soy's potential for protecting women against breast cancer – and another reason to boost the soya content of your diet if you haven't already done so. In a recent issue of *Cancer Epidemiology, Biomarkers & Prevention*, it was claimed that regular consumption of soy-based foods was associated with lower levels of the hormone oestrone. Oestrone is the form of oestrogen that is predominant following menopause, and which is associated with elevated breast cancer risk.

In Singapore, a group of 144 healthy Chinese women between the ages of 50 and 74, were interviewed in detail about their diet (particularly in relation to 165 specific food items), reproductive history and various lifestyle factors.

Six types of soy foods and one soy drink were included in the food items, and total soy as well as soy isoflavone intake was calculated. Blood samples were then analysed for levels of oestrogens.

Soy emerged as the one dietary factor that was associated with lower levels of oestrone.

When isoflavone consumption was examined, high levels were also found to be associated with lower serum oestrone.

The lead investigator and Professor of Preventive Medicine at the Keck School of Medicine at the University of Southern California, Anna H. Wu, said: "Results from this study support the hypothesis that high soy intake may reduce the risk of breast cancer by lowering endogenous oestrogen levels, particularly oestrone."

There are many delicious soy-based foods to choose from – in the form of soy milk, yoghurts and tofu – all available in supermarkets and health food stores. Miso, used for stock and soups, is made from fermented soya beans – try the healthy and delicious miso soup recipe on page 113.

How to benefit from hemp seed's perfect balance of omega-3 and omega-6 fatty acids

The nutritional benefits of hemp seed are also noteworthy, particularly in the form of hemp seed oil, and are mainly due to its perfect balance of omega-6 and omega-3 EFAs. Hemp seed oil also contains substantial amounts of gamma-linolenic acid (GLA), which is the only edible seed to do so. GLA is a polyunsaturated fatty acid that can be produced in the body from linoleic acid. However, those with premenstrual syndrome, diabetes, scleroderma, Sjogren's syndrome, eczema and other skin conditions are thought to have a metabolic block that interferes with the body's ability to make GLA. In preliminary research, supplementation with GLA has helped sufferers of these conditions.

Many people in Western societies may be at least partially GLA-deficient as a result of ageing, glucose intolerance, dietary fat intake, and other problems. Due to hemp seed oil being a rich source of GLA it is particularly beneficial as an alternative to other GLA rich sources such as starflower or evening primrose oil.

Hemp seed oil, like other polyunsaturated fats, is inherently unstable, and can react to heat, light or oxygen to form unhealthy molecules (free radicals). Therefore it is vital to obtain hemp seed oil that has been processed under strict conditions, and stored in opaque bottles in a refrigerator. Hemp seed oil should never be heated or used in cooking. It is best added to salads or grains – approximately one tablespoon (15ml) a day. Benefits from taking hemp seed oil normally start to show after about four to six weeks of use. Regular users report that only after a few weeks their skin feels softer, nails become stronger and hair becomes shinier.

Salba seeds – This Aztec staple can help overcome everything from constipation to high blood sugar levels

Salba seeds – even though chia might have seemed like an unlikely super food 25 years ago, none of the grain's health perks were discovered by accident. In fact, it has a history as a nutritive staple for warriors and hunters of the Aztec civilization. Not only did the seeds sustain them on long expeditions, but they also played a role in many of the culture's holy ceremonies as well.

It was such a powerful element of this ancient society that, on the heels of the Spanish invasion of Mexico in the 16th century, Conquistadors set out to burn every last chia crop to the ground – a strategy they viewed as essential to their ultimate conquest of the territory. But despite being a victim of these historical events chia has been granted another incarnation as Salba.

Salba is carefully cultivated on farms in Peru and other South American locations to ensure nutritional consistency – and because of these controlled factors, the seed typically has a much higher omega-3 and protein content than its earlier version.

As you can imagine, these advances serve to bolster the fact that chia – and especially the patented Salba – makes for stiff competition against flaxseed when it comes to a convenient plant-based source of protein, fibre and alpha-linolenic acid. Just to put that into perspective: two tablespoons contains more fibre than a serving of the constipation remedy Metamucil and delivers 3,050mg of omega-3s – that's the equivalent of more than five flax oil capsules, or 10 fish oil capsules.

Salba's comparison charts are striking. But there's one thing that you should bear in mind – and this caveat applies to flaxseed as well. Linolenic acid's true value to your body only takes shape after it's converted into eicosapentaenoic acid (EPA) and docosahexaenoic acid (DHA).

It's these latter fatty acids specifically (which are already formed in food sources such as salmon and other cold-water fish) that are known to boost the production of the prostaglandins that mediate inflammation, clotting mechanisms and cardiovascular health.

Unfortunately, the conversion rate of linolenic acid into EPA and DHA within the human body is thought to be relatively low, which means that using plants as your primary source of omega-3s may not always be sufficient. So while Salba's loaded with a lot of great nutrition – including plenty of alpha-linolenic acid – if you're taking fish oil supplements, you'll probably want to continue taking them in order to get the maximum benefits of a diet that's rich in essential fatty acids.

But that's not to say that Salba doesn't have its advantages over fish oil, too. It also contains lots of other vitamins and minerals. These include calcium, iron, copper, magnesium, potassium, phosphorus, zinc, molybdenum, and vitamins A, B and C. The seeds' antioxidant content is equally impressive – including myricetin, kaempferol and quercetin.

Probably the most important on this list are chlorogenic and caffeic acid – two compounds which aid glucose metabolism and weight control (*Weber, C.W. 1991. "The nutritional and chemical evaluation of chia seeds." Ecology of Food and Nutrition 26: 119-125*). But it's all of these powerful antioxidants working together that protects Salba from going rancid quickly – which, as mentioned earlier, is one of flax's more notorious tendencies.

The first of two small studies conducted by a Canadian research team at the University of Toronto examined the postprandial glycemic responses of six healthy fasting men between the ages of 39 and 44.

Each of the six were fed either a standardized portion of white bread consisting of 50 grams of available carbohydrate, or the same portion of another bread prepared with 30 grams of Salba. The subjects who ate the Salba-enriched bread experienced less extreme fluctuations in blood glucose levels at both 60 and 120 minutes after consumption

(*Bazinet R, Sievenpiper J, Stavro M, et al. "Salvia hispanica l. seed is a rich source of alpha-linolenic acid and prolongs postprandial glycemia." Faculty of Medicine, Department of Nutritional Sciences, University of Toronto*).

The second pilot study began by assessing the glucose, cholesterol, and triglyceride (blood fat) levels of two subjects, who then began supplementing with 50 grams of Salba per day. After two weeks, results showed that Salba had a positive effect on all of the measured factors – meaning that it might be an essential tool in maintaining healthy lipid levels and minimizing cardiovascular risk.

Another larger single-blind study conducted by Salba's manufacturers tracked the effects of Salba supplementation on a group of 20 individuals – each of which received either Salba or a control supplement for a period of 12 weeks. Results showed that Salba may help to control the production of both C-reactive protein and fibrinogen, thereby promoting healthy inflammation responses and normal clotting mechanisms in the blood.

It's true that none of these studies were very long, nor did they follow a substantial group of subjects. Nevertheless, the initial results of these pilot studies are extremely promising – and in all likelihood, just a preview of what's to come in the years ahead.

The taste of Salba seeds is barely detectable – at most they have a faint cucumber-like flavour (which would definitely be masked by just about any recipe in which you might choose to use them).

To any given amount of seeds, add four times as much water (e.g. two tablespoons of the seed for each half-cup of water), and the result will be a nutrition-packed, near-flavourless gel that you can add to yoghurt or porridge, or use as a spread on toast.

Fill up on these nutritious seeds and pulses too

You should eat more lentils too. Just one cooked cup of these beneficial pulses contain 17 grams of protein, a whopping 8 grams of fibre (about a third of the daily value), more than 35 per cent of your iron and potassium needs and 175 per cent of the RDA for a B vitamin called folate. Recent research shows that folate is crucial for maintaining overall good health; the nutrient is essential for the production of new cells, especially the millions of blood cells created by your body daily (*Br J Nutr. 1999 Sep; 82(3): 203-12*). Try making the 'comforting lentil and tomato soup' recipe on the next page – it provides a hearty and nutritious meal when it's cold outside.

Pumpkin seeds may help maintain prostate health in men. Studies performed at Vienna University have revealed that swelling of the prostate is almost non-existent among men in Transylvania. Research conducted in the Transylvanian Alps has hinted that this phenomenon may be attributed to the Transylvanian passion for pumpkin seeds. Pumpkin seeds contain large amounts of magnesium, which French physicians have proven to be effective in the treatment of prostate ailments. The seeds are also an excellent source of zinc, which has also been linked to good prostate health.

Sesame seeds – containing no less than eight nutrients – help prevent infertility, raise sexual drive and improve overall health. They are one of the highest sources of the trace element selenium, essential for optimum immunity – and a higher sperm count. Grind the seeds in a blender before eating them to release their mineral content.

Comforting lentil and tomato soup

This recipe serves 4 people

For this dish you will need the following ingredients:

2 x 400g tins green lentils
1x 400g can of chopped tomatoes
2 tbsp of tomato purée
1 litre vegetable stock
2 tbsp extra virgin olive oil
1 onion (chopped)
2-3 garlic cloves (crushed)
2 tsp ground coriander
1 tbsp ground cumin
Natural yogurt, fresh coriander and toasted pitta bread, to serve

To prepare:

Heat the oil in a large saucepan. Add the onions and garlic and cook until soft. Add the coriander and cumin and cook, stirring, for two minutes.

Add the tomatoes, purée, stock and season. Bring to the boil, then reduce heat slightly and add the lentils. Simmer rapidly for 20 minutes until slightly reduced, thickened and piping hot. Serve with some natural yogurt, fresh coriander and toasted wholemeal pitta bread cut into slices.

Hearty split pea soup

This recipe serves 6 people

For this dish you will need the following ingredients:

375g of split green or yellow peas (soaked for at least 4 hours)
1 large onion (finely chopped)
2 large carrots (finely chopped)
2 celery sticks (finely chopped)
2 crushed garlic cloves
1 bay leaf
3 sprigs of fresh parsley
1 sprig of fresh thyme
1.5 litres of chicken or vegetable stock
Salt and pepper
6 tbsp of thick Greek-style yoghurt to serve (optional)

To prepare:

Drain the split peas and transfer them into a large saucepan with all the herbs and vegetables. Season with salt and pepper and add enough stock to cover the contents by about 1 inch. Bring to the boil and boil for 10 minutes and then simmer gently for about one to one and a half hours until the peas have become a rough purée. Stir occasionally and add extra water if the soup becomes too thick. Remove the thyme and parsley sprigs and the bay leaf. Serve while hot and add a tablespoon of the Greek-style yoghurt to each bowl.

Tuna and butter bean salad

This recipe serves 4 people

For this dish you will need the following ingredients:

3 tbsp of extra virgin olive oil
1 tbsp of white wine vinegar
½ tsp of sugar
½ tsp of Dijon mustard
Salt and pepper
425g can butter beans (drained)
3 large cans of tuna fish in spring water (drained and flaked)

Chopped capers to garnish

To prepare:

Put the olive oil, vinegar, mustard and sugar in a large bowl and season with salt and pepper. Stir well. In another bowl put in the tuna and butter beans and mix well. Pour the dressing over the tuna and butter bean mix and toss well. Put into a serving dish and garnish with capers. You may prefer to eat this on a bed of lettuce.

Mushroom and miso soup

This recipe serves 5 people

For this dish you will need the following ingredients:

3 tbs miso
100g firm tofu, cut in 1 cm cubes
100g mushrooms, sliced
2 tbs dashi (from Asian shop)
1 litre of vegetable stock
2 stalks green onions, chopped

To prepare:

Boil the stock and add the dashi, mushrooms and tofu squares. Simmer for approximately five minutes. Then add and dissolve the miso.

Just before serving sprinkle over the green onions. For best results serve the mushroom and miso soup hot.

Chickpea casserole with spinach

This recipe serves 2 people

For this dish you will need the following ingredients:

2-3 tbsp extra virgin olive oil
1 red onion, roughly chopped
2 cloves of garlic, finely sliced
½ tsp ground coriander
½ tsp black mustard seeds
1 tin (400g) chickpeas, liquid included
1 potato, cut into small chunks
1 red pepper, deseeded, cut into 8 strips
125g (half a bag) washed baby spinach
2 tomatoes, quartered
2 tbsp soy sauce
1 small red chilli, finely chopped
salt and pepper
Live natural yoghurt
Lemon wedges
Wholemeal pitta breads

To prepare:

Heat the olive oil in a large saucepan over a medium heat and then add the red onion, garlic and chilli and sweat until transparent. Add the ground coriander and the mustard seeds and fry for a minute or so, adding 1 or 2 tbsp liquid from the tin of chickpeas.

Add the chopped potato and stir in until well coated with the spices. Allow to cook for five or six minutes until the potatoes are almost soft. Then add the chickpeas and the rest of the liquid and simmer gently for five to seven minutes until the sauce is thick and rich.

Meanwhile, heat your griddle pan and sauté the red pepper strips in the remaining oil until charred in places. Add to the chickpeas then gently add in the baby spinach and stir until wilted.

Add the tomato quarters and cook until just soft. Finish with the soy sauce and extra olive oil if you like.

Serve with a bowl of natural live yoghurt and some lemon wedges too, as well as some toasted pitta breads.

CHAPTER 5

Herbs and spices add flavour and health-promoting properties to your food

The health benefits linked to herbs and spices is well-known, particularly in Traditional Chinese Medicine. Some of the best ones include:

Basil: A simple way to maintain the health of your heart

Want to enrich the taste and cardiovascular health benefits of your pasta sauce? Add a good helping of basil (*Ocimum basilicum*). The herb is a good source of magnesium, which promotes cardiovascular health by prompting muscles and blood vessels to relax, thereby improving blood flow and lessening the risk of irregular heart rhythms or a spasming of the heart muscle or a blood vessel.

Basil also helps maintain the health of your heart as a result of its high amounts of vitamin A (through its concentration of carotenoids such as beta-carotene), which not only protects epithelial cells (the cells that form the lining of numerous body structures including the blood vessels) from free radical damage, but also helps prevent free radicals from oxidizing cholesterol in the bloodstream. Only after it has been oxidized does cholesterol build up in blood vessel walls, initiating the development of atherosclerosis, whose end result can be a heart attack or stroke.

Free radical damage is a contributing factor in many other conditions as well, including asthma, osteoarthritis, and rheumatoid arthritis. The beta-carotene found in basil may help to lessen the progression of these conditions while protecting cells from further damage.

It is also a very good source of iron, calcium, potassium and vitamin C.

Basil helps fight drug-resistant strains of bacteria

The unique array of active constituents called flavonoids found in basil provide protection at the cellular level. Orientin and vicenin are two water-soluble flavonoids that have been of particular interest in basil, and in studies on human white blood cells, these components of basil protect cell structures as well as chromosomes from radiation and oxygen-based damage.

The volatile oils it contains possess potent antibacterial properties and studies have demonstrated that it is effective at restricting the growth of numerous bacteria, including: *Listeria monocytogenes, Staphylococcus aureus, Escherichia coli* O:157:H7, *Yersinia enterocolitica,* and *Pseudomonas aeruginosa.*

Essential oil of basil, obtained from its leaves, has demonstrated the ability to inhibit several species of pathogenic bacteria that have become resistant to commonly used antibiotic drugs.

In a study published in the July 2003 issue of the *Journal of Microbiology Methods,* essential oil of basil was even found to inhibit strains of bacteria from the genera *Staphylococcus, Enterococcus* and *Pseudomonas* – all of which are not only widespread, but now pose serious treatment difficulties because they have developed a high level of resistance to treatment with antibiotic drugs.

Basil provides effective relief from swelling

The eugenol component of basil's volatile oils has been the subject of extensive study, since this substance can block the activity of an inflammatory enzyme in the body called cyclooxygenase (COX).

Many non-steriodal, over-the-counter, anti-inflammatory medications (NSAIDS), including aspirin and ibuprofen, as well as the commonly used medicine acetaminophen, work by inhibiting this same enzyme but all come with a long list of harmful side effects.

This enzyme-inhibiting effect of the eugenol in basil qualifies basil as an 'anti-inflammatory' food that can provide important healing benefits along with symptomatic relief for sufferers of inflammatory health problems like rheumatoid arthritis or inflammatory bowel conditions.

Cod in tomato and basil sauce

This recipe serves 4 people

For this dish you will need the following ingredients:

8 large basil leaves
4 skinless cod fillets
1 onion (finely chopped)
1 small aubergine (chopped)
1 tbsp of extra virgin olive oil
½ tsp ground paprika
2 cloves of garlic (crushed)
400g can of chopped tomatoes
1 tsp light or dark muscovado sugar

To prepare:

Stir-fry the aubergine and onion in the extra virgin olive oil for five minutes. Cover with a lid and let the veg steam for six minutes. Stir in the paprika, garlic, tomatoes and sugar with some seasoning and simmer for a further 10 minutes, stirring until the onion and aubergine are tender.

Scatter in the basil leaves then place the fish in the sauce, cover the pan and simmer for approximately 10 minutes, or until cooked.

Cinnamon: Discover how an ordinary kitchen spice led to the development of an extraordinary diabetes remedy

Cinnamon, the dried inner bark of a tree from Sri Lanka, is a common ingredient used to flavour a variety of dishes that you probably have sitting on your kitchen spice rack.

Latest research findings have revealed that this popular spice possesses far more than a distinctive taste. It is proving to have remarkable powers as a safe and effective treatment for diabetes.

In 1990, Dr Richard Anderson, a chemist at the Human Nutrition Research Center in Maryland, in the US, was searching for foods that might mimic the action of insulin in controlling blood sugar. He was amazed to discover that the spice mix used in the traditional American apple pie had just this effect, which was finally narrowed down to its content of cinnamon.

Diabetes can cause additional complications... as can conventional diabetes drugs

Diabetes causes blood sugar levels to become damagingly high because the hormone insulin is not regulating it properly. In Type 1 diabetes, which usually becomes apparent in childhood, the pancreas (a gland situated behind your stomach) produces little or no insulin. This usually requires daily injections of insulin.

In the kind of diabetes that most often arises in later life, called Type 2, either the system that signals the pancreas to produce insulin becomes less efficient or the body tissues become less responsive to insulin – a condition called insulin resistance.

Common symptoms of Type 2 diabetes are fatigue, frequent hunger, excessive thirst and a frequent need to urinate. It can also cause blurred vision, a dry mouth and dry or itchy skin. It is important to see your doctor immediately if you suspect you may be developing diabetes, as it can be a life-threatening condition. If not well controlled, the long-term effects of diabetes can lead to heart disease, stroke, kidney failure, vision loss and nerve damage.

While conventional anti-diabetic drugs like Metformin can control blood sugar levels effectively, they come with a long list of harmful side effects, including dizziness, fatigue, headaches, nervousness, confusion, nausea, sweating and loss of appetite.

Clinical trials involving diabetic patients and cinnamon have revealed startling results

It was 13 years after Dr Anderson's initial discovery that cinnamon can successfully control blood sugar levels, that a research associate of his, Dr Alam Khan, leading a team at the Hayatabad Medical Complex in Peshawar, Pakistan, conducted a clinical trial in diabetes patients.

Sixty middle-aged men and women were divided into groups who received either 1, 3 or 6 grams of powdered cinnamon daily, or a placebo. After 40 days, patients in all three of the cinnamon groups had reductions in their blood sugar levels of between 18 and 29 per cent, while there was no change in the placebo group (*Diabetes Care 2003; 26(12): 3215-3218*).

This trial was carried out in Pakistan and the patients' diabetes was not under the degree of control that would be typically aimed for in the West, so their blood sugar levels at the start of the trial were relatively high by comparison. The patients' diets and genetic backgrounds were also different from those of most Westerners. Because of this, it was still not certain that cinnamon would be an effective addition to conventional medical treatments for diabetes.

Now, cutting-edge new research from Germany has removed any remaining doubts about cinnamon's effectiveness. A team at the University of Hannover conducted a double-blind clinical trial in which 79 patients with Type 2 diabetes were given either an aqueous cinnamon extract (equivalent to 3 grams powdered cinnamon) or a placebo capsule, three times a day for four months (*Eur J Clin Invest 2006; 36(5): 340-344*).

At the end of the trial, blood sugar levels had fallen by an average of 10 per cent in the group taking cinnamon extract, but by only 3 per cent in the control group. The patients who had the highest blood sugar readings at the start of the trial experienced the greatest reductions. This explains why the results of the German trial, while being comparable with the effects of conventional medication, were not as spectacular as those in Pakistan, where patients were starting from much higher blood sugar level readings.

Boosts insulin activity and increases glucose metabolism

Cinnamon contains two main active ingredients. One of these is a group of water-soluble compounds called polyphenols, which promote glucose uptake by cells and increase glucose metabolism. The most important polyphenol it contains is MHCP, which boosts the activity of insulin by about 20 times (*J Agric Food Chem 2004; 52: 65-70*).

The other active ingredient is a group of compounds known as hydroxychalcones, which actually mimic the action of insulin and allow glucose to pass from the bloodstream into the cells (*J Am Coll Nutr 2001; 20(4): 327-336*).

Quick and delicious banana and cinnamon smoothie

This recipe serves 1-2 people

For this dish you will need the following ingredients:

1 large pinch of ground cinnamon
1 banana (cut into chunks)
150g pot of live natural yoghurt
150ml semi-skimmed milk
1 tsp honey

To prepare:

Chop the banana into large chunks and place the banana, milk, live yoghurt, honey and cinnamon into a blender and blend until smooth. Pour into a glass and serve with a little extra cinnamon sprinkled over the top.

Fennel: Far more than a simple recipe ingredient... it helps fight everything from infections to obesity

In many parts of Asia it is customary to chew on fennel seeds (which taste very similar to liquorice) following a meal, in order to freshen the breath and aid digestion. In addition to the seeds, other parts of the fennel (*Foeniculum vulgare*) plant – including the bulb, stalk and leaves – are used for culinary purposes across the globe. For example, in both France and Italy fennel is considered to be one of the best herbs to add to fish dishes, and it is also used to flavour breads, cakes and confectionery.

Fennel also has a long history of use as a medicinal herb for alleviating a diverse range of ailments – including persistent coughs, stomach problems, sinusitis, colic and menstrual cramps. Research is now verifying its use in many of these areas.

For example, Iranian scientists from the Department of Obstetrics and Gynaecology, Kerman University of Medical Sciences and Health Services, found that fennel extracts are more effective at relieving period pain than the conventional treatment mefenamic acid (also known as Ponstan).

The scientists divided two groups of teenage girls, all of whom suffered from extremely painful periods each month, and gave them either fennel extract or mefenamic acid. They found that 80 per cent of the girls who received fennel experienced complete pain relief compared to 73 per cent of those taking mefenamic acid (*Modaress Nejad V, Asadipour M. East Mediterr Health J. 2006; 12(3-4): 423-7*). Better still, fennel has no adverse effects whereas mefenamic acid can cause diarrhoea, nausea and vomiting.

As well as backing up some of fennel's traditional uses, ongoing research is revealing additional therapeutic benefits attached to the herb. This is hardly surprising given the numerous medicinal properties it contains, including the free-radical fighting antioxidants estragole, flavonoids, quercetin and rutin. It also contains a compound called anethole, which is known to act as an oestrogen stimulant – increasing milk production, promoting menstruation and reducing symptoms of the male menopause such as lowered libido, fatigue and mood swings.

Fennel's diverse list of therapeutic actions just keeps on growing

According to the latest research findings fennel acts as a memory booster. In an animal study, scientists at the Department of Pharmacognosy, SET's College of Pharmacy, Karnataka, in India, studied the effects of fennel on age-related memory loss associated with dementia.

The scientists found that mice receiving fennel supplements were able to remember several tasks far better than mice who did not receive any treatment. Commenting on the findings the scientists concluded that: "Fennel can be employed in the treatment of cognitive disorders such as dementia and Alzheimer's disease" (*Joshi H, Parle M. J Med Food. 2006; 9(3): 413-7*).

Another area in which fennel is showing a great deal of promise is against infections. In fact, it has been found to help combat several different types of infection. Research published just a few weeks ago by Turkish scientists working at the Department of Food Engineering, Selcuk University, revealed that fennel is effective against bacteria that cause food poisoning (*Ozcan MM, Sagdic O, Ozkan G. J Med Food. 2006 Fall; 9(3): 418-21*). Separate research has shown that it can also help combat salmonella, thrush and infective diarrhoea (*Khaldun AO. Zh Mikrobiol Epidemiol Immunobiol. 2006 May-Jun; (3): 92-3*).

Scientists have also discovered that fennel extracts have anti-inflammatory properties, and can help alleviate joint pain and allergic reactions. It is thought that fennel helps protect your tissues against toxic chemicals like glutamate and nitric oxide, which are produced during the inflammation process. It also appears to work in the brain to reduce feelings of pain (*Fitoterapia. 2004 Sep; 75(6): 557-65*).

How fennel can help in the battle of the bulge

Fennel's numerous beneficial actions don't end there. New research suggests that it can also help prevent weight gain through controlling appetite. An animal study conducted at the Thuringian State Institute of Agriculture, Jena, in Germany found that including more fennel in the diet significantly reduced overall food intake (*Schone F, et al. J Anim Physiol Anim Nutr (Berl). 2006 Dec; 90(11-12): 500-10*).

In a separate animal study conducted at the School of Nursing, Eulji University, in Korea, scientists set out to determine if inhaling aromatic oils from several plants had any effect on body weight or appetite. Three groups of rats were given aromatherapy oils to inhale from fennel, patchouli and bergamot respectively, while a fourth group was used for comparison only.

The treatment was applied for 10 minutes twice a day for eight weeks. At the end of the study the scientists found that the rats treated with fennel were better able to digest food, in addition to assimilating less calories from it, compared to the other groups (*Hur MH, Kim C, Kim CH, Ahn HC, Ahn HY. Taehan Kanho Hakhoe Chi. 2006 Apr; 36(2): 236-43*).

Fresh fennel and walnut salad

This recipe serves 2 people

For this dish you will need the following ingredients:

4 small fennel bulbs (cored and thinly sliced)
2 tomatoes (cut into quarters)
2 spring onions (sliced)
1 small cucumber (sliced)
1 avocado (sliced)
50g walnuts (chopped)
100g green olives
3 tbsp of extra virgin olive oil
1 tbsp of white wine vinegar
1 garlic clove (crushed)
1 tbsp of fresh parsley (chopped)
1 tbsp of fresh dill (chopped)
Salt and pepper

To prepare:

Mix the oil, vinegar, garlic, salt, pepper, dill and parsley in a bowl. Add the fennel, avocado, olives, spring onions, tomatoes, cucumber and walnuts to the bowl and toss well.

Ginger: The spice with a diverse range of therapeutic actions

Studies are revealing that ginger is an effective remedy for alleviating arthritis pain. Gingers contains many anti-inflammatory chemicals which block several pathways to the destruction of cartilage (*Pharmacol 1994,49(5) 314-318*).

Ginger is also very effective for alleviating nausea and regulating digestive functioning. The spice has long been reputed to have medicinal properties: in India, ginger tea is touted as a remedy for the common cold.

Exciting new research findings recently presented at the 2003 American Association for Cancer Research's Second Annual International Conference on Frontiers in Cancer Prevention Research, have revealed that ginger shows a great deal of promise in the fight against colorectal (bowel) cancer.

Although these findings are based on an animal study, they are potentially very promising as this disease is second only to lung cancer in being the most common cause of cancer deaths in the UK. The statistics make scary reading – each year in the UK approximately 35,000 people are diagnosed with bowel cancer and 16,00 people die from it. So any formula that can help prevent or treat the disease is desperately needed.

The study was carried out by scientists from the University of

Minnesota's Hormel Institute in Austin, Minnesota in the US. They found that 6-gingerol – a compound found in ginger that gives the spice its distinct flavour – was able to significantly slow the growth of colorectal cancer cells in mice, compared to those that didn't receive any treatment.

Dr Ann Bode, Associate Professor of Research at the University of Minnesota's Hormel Institute, who was part of the team that carried out the study, said: "The results strongly suggest that ginger compounds may slow the growth of cancers or reduce the size of established tumours". Adding: "Plants of the ginger family have been credited with therapeutic and preventive powers and have been reported to have anti-cancer activity... These results strongly suggest that ginger compounds may be effective chemo-preventive and/or chemotherapeutic agents for colorectal carcinomas."

Further studies are now being planned to look into ginger's potential anti-cancer action in the area of bowel cancer.

To benefit, include plenty of fresh ginger in your diet – you can chop it up and add it to your meals to add flavour or make it into a pleasant-tasting drink simply by adding boiling water.

Prawn and veggie ginger stir-fry

This recipe serves 2 people

For this dish you will need the following ingredients:

350g of prawns (shelled)
2 leeks (finely chopped)
1 tbsp of extra virgin olive oil
1cm piece of fresh root ginger, peeled and finely chopped
1-2 garlic cloves (crushed or chopped finely)
125g of button mushrooms (cut into quarters)
50g of bean sprouts

1 tbsp of soy sauce
1 tsp of sesame oil
Pepper

To prepare:

Heat the oil in a wok or large frying pan over a medium to high heat. Add the ginger and garlic, stir, then add the leeks and stir-fry for one minute. Add the bean sprouts and continue stir-frying for a further minute. Add the mushrooms, sesame oil, prawns and soy sauce, and continue to stir-fry for three to four minutes or until the prawns are pink and just cooked through. Season with pepper and serve immediately.

Instant energy ginger juice

This drink serves 1 person

For this drink you will need the following ingredients:

2 apples (quartered)
3 carrots (chopped)
2.5cm of fresh root ginger (finely chopped)
Ice cubes (to serve)

To prepare:

Simply put the apples, carrots and ginger into a juicer (or blender) and stir well. Pour into a glass with plenty of ice and drink.

Oregano: The herb that's generating a great deal of excitement in the scientific community for its ability to treat everything from urinary to fungal infections

Oregano (*Origanum vulgare*) is usually thought of as a culinary herb used primarily in Italian, Greek and Mediterranean cooking, but it has also been used for many centuries as a medicinal plant.

Traditionally, oregano oil has been used to treat a wide range of conditions from urinary infections, asthma and coughs to indigestion, diarrhoea and vomiting. The ancient Greeks were among the first to take advantage of its curative qualities, and made compresses from the leaves to treat sores and aching muscles.

However, it has only been recently that scientists have taken an interest in the herb's medicinal properties, and evidence is now in the process of being gathered which backs up many of its traditional therapeutic uses and also reveals additional benefits linked to the herb.

With regards to the latter, oregano has been found to contain several powerful antioxidants – such as phenolic acids and flavonoids – which protect your tissues against harmful toxins like cancer-causing free radicals (*Tian H, Lai DM. Zhong Yao Cai. 2006; 29(9): 920-1; Hazzit M, et al. J Agric Food Chem. 2006; 54(17): 6314-21*).

In fact, oregano was found to come up tops in another related study conducted by Canadian scientists from the University of Quebec. The researchers compared several herbs, including cinnamon and sage, in terms of their ability to fight harmful chemicals, such as free radicals and nitric oxide, which are known to increase the risk of chronic diseases like arthritis, heart disease, dementia and cancer. The oregano extracts were found to possess by far the strongest activity against these harmful toxins (*Salmieri S, Lacroix M.: J Agric Food Chem. 2006 Dec 27; 54(26): 10205-14*).

Scientists confirm what many traditional healers have known for centuries

With regards to evidence backing up oregano's traditional medicinal uses, the area that has received the most attention by scientists to date, relates to the herb's ability to combat infections.

Scientists have discovered that its benefits for alleviating urinary tract infections are mainly a result of its powerful anti-inflammatory properties – oregano contains an active ingredient called rosmarinic acid that is known to inhibit inflammation.

In addition, Greek scientists from the Department of Pharmacognosy and Chemistry of Natural Products, University of Athens, have found that essential oils from oregano contain a substance called carvacrol, which is also able to prevent inflammatory processes from taking place in the body (*Karioti A, Vrahimi-Hadjilouca T, et al. Planta Med. 2006 Nov; 72(14): 1330-4*).

The herb has also been found to act as a powerful fungicide and can be used to treat fungus and yeast infections like thrush, which is caused by a yeast overgrowth.

Oregano's infection-fighting benefits extend to protecting against food poisoning

Japanese scientists from the National Research Institute of Fisheries Science in Yokohama, have reported that oregano can block the growth of an infectious bug called *Vibrio parahaemolyticus*, which contaminates food and can cause food poisoning (*Yano Y, Satomi M, Oikawa H. Int J Food Microbiol. 2006 Aug 15; 111(1): 6-11*).

In addition, researchers from the Agricultural Faculty, Selcuk University in Turkey studied essential oils from several different plants, including oregano, laurel, marjoram and mint. They tested these oils on certain bacteria (including *Bacillus*, which can cause bowel infections and diarrhoea) in the laboratory. All of the herbs, including oregano, were found to successfully block the growth of the bacteria studied (*Ozcan MM, Sagdic O, Ozkan G. J Med Food. 2006 Fall; 9(3): 418-21*).

In an animal study, performed by scientists at the National Agricultural Research Foundation in Greece, oregano was found to be just as effective as the prescription-only antibiotic neomycin for curing diarrhoea caused by the *E.coli* bug, which is notorious for causing bowel infections.

Commenting on the findings the scientists said: "This study indicates that dried oregano leaves may be as effective in the treatment of coli infection as neomycin" (*Bampidis VA, et al. J Vet Med A Physiol Pathol Clin Med. 2006; 53(3): 154-6*). This finding is important because it indicates that oregano extracts could prove to be a safe and effective alternative to antibiotics, which can cause several unpleasant side effects including vomiting, allergic rash, and – ironically – diarrhoea.

Scientists believe that one way oregano successfully fights infections is by destroying the protective outer shell of the infectious bacteria. Another theory is that it may work by interrupting the energy supply to the bacteria, so starving them to death. But it is likely that there are many other mechanisms by which oregano works, which still need to be investigated.

How to take advantage of oregano's healing powers

Dried oregano herb can be mixed with boiling water to make a tea, which can then be drunk two or three times a day.

You can also take advantage of the herb's anti-inflammatory properties to relieve tired joints and muscles by putting a handful of oregano leaves in a coffee filter, mesh bag, or cheesecloth bag and running steaming bath water over it. Allow it to steep in the tub with you as you relax in the warm, fragrant water.

In Cass Ingram's book *Supermarket Remedies*, he states that 'oregano is one of Nature's finest preservatives'. He suggests that if oregano is used with foods such as meat, eggs, milk, or salad, you 'will greatly halt the growth of microbes and, thus, reduce the risk of food poisoning'.

Black olives with oregano

For this dish you will need the following ingredients:

1lb black olives
3-4 cloves of garlic, thinly sliced
1 tbsp oregano
2 tbsp vinegar
8 tbsp extra virgin olive oil

To prepare:

Place the olives in a bowl and add all the ingredients. Stir well and allow to marinate overnight before serving.

Rosemary: The well-known herb with hidden benefits... including an ability to prevent cancer

Rosemary (*Rosmarinus officinalis*) is a well-known culinary herb. Dried rosemary leaves, whole or ground, are a popular seasoning for food... adding flavour to soups, stews, meat and fish.

Applied to the skin, rosemary essential oil helps strengthen the capillaries and has a rejuvenating effect. For this reason, rosemary is a common ingredient used in many cosmetics, including skin toners, creams, soaps and hair products.

However, beyond being a flavouring-enhancer for certain foods and its use in cosmetics, you may not be aware that rosemary extract has a long history of medicinal uses too. It has been used to treat a wide range of ailments, including stomach upset, digestive disorders, headaches, and renal colic (sudden pain caused by kidney stones in the ureter).

Recent research is now revealing even more benefits attached to this remarkable herb, including its ability to help prevent cancer and age-related skin damage, boost the functioning of the liver and act as mild diuretic to help reduce swelling.

Two of the most important ingredients in rosemary, which are thought to be largely responsible for many of these therapeutic actions, are caffeic acid and rosmarinic acid – both are potent antioxidant and anti-inflammatory agents (*Masuda T et al. J Agric Food Chem 2002; 50(21): 5863-5869*). These two natural acids are effective at reducing inflammation which may contribute to asthma, liver disease and heart disease (*al-Sereiti MR et al. Indian J Exp Biol 1999; 37(2): 124-130*).

Rosemary is proving an important defence against cancer

The antioxidants contained in rosemary help to protect your body's cells from free radicals attack. They include monoterpenes, phenolic diterpenes and flavonoids, which are renowned for their ability to slow down the production of free radicals (*Saen-Lopez R et al. J Chromatogr A 2002953(1-2): 251-256; Lee KG, Shibamoto T. J Agric Food Chem 2002; 50(17): 4947-4952*). It is also a rich source of vitamin E (alpha tocopherol), another potent antioxidant, which contributes to its free radical fighting powers further still (*Torre J et al. J Chromatogr A 2001; 919(2): 305-311*).

DNA is your genetic blueprint, and it is particularly prone to injury caused by free radicals. Left unchecked, this damage can eventually lead to cells proliferating out of control, which greatly increases the risk of cancer.

Scientists from the department of Mutagenesis and Carcinogenesis, Cancer Research Institute of Slovak Academy of Sciences, in the Slovak Republic, have found that rosemary extract can significantly help to protect DNA against free radical damage (*Slamenova D et al. Cancer Lett 2002; 177(2): 145-153*).

By blocking oestrogen, rosemary helps prevent against breast cancer

It is well known that an imbalance of oestrogen hormones in women can contribute to breast cancer and cancer of the uterus. Several conventional drugs such as tamoxifen are aimed at blocking the effects of oestrogen to help reduce this risk. However, tamoxifen can cause a range of unpleasant side effects, including hot flushes, vaginal bleeding, headaches and nausea.

Fortunately, rosemary offers a safe and natural alternative treatment. Dr Zhu and colleagues from the Department of Chemical Biology, State University of New Jersey in the US, found that a 2 per cent concentration of rosemary extract given for three weeks was able to significantly inactivate excess oestrogen. Researchers believe that it works by stimulating liver enzymes, which inactivate oestrogen hormones like oestrone and oestradiol (*Zhu BT et al. Carcinogenesis 1998: 19(10): 1821-1827*).

Rosemary helps minimise the effects of ageing on your skin

As mentioned earlier, one of the traditional uses of rosemary is as a cosmetic. Recent research findings have now confirmed the skin-protective benefits it possesses.

According to researchers working at the Faculty of Medicine, University of Catania, in Italy, rosemary extract helps protect the individual components of skin cells, including the cell membrane, which may prevent age-related skin damage, such as wrinkles (*Calabrese V et al. Int J Tissue React 2000; 22(1): 5-13*).

In a follow-up study the Italian researchers found that rosemary extract is able to exert even greater benefits. In particular, it was shown to safeguard a protective protein called HsP70. The role of this protein is to reduce damage caused by stress, free radicals and other toxins on the skin (*Calabrese V et al. Int J Tissue React 2001; 23(2): 51-58*).

Disarms harmful toxins and flushes them from your body

Another benefit rosemary extract has been shown to possess is an ability to inactivate toxins and then eliminate them from your liver, before they can inflict any serious damage.

French scientists from the National Institute of Agronomic Research in Dijon, found that rosemary extract encouraged detoxifying enzymes – including cytochrome P450 glutathione transferase and quinone reductase – to flush harmful toxins from the liver (*Debersac P et al. Food Chem Toxicol 2001: 39(9): 907-918*).

In effect, rosemary stimulates your liver to work more efficiently. By stimulating your liver to eliminate any impurities in your blood, it helps you feel more healthy and energetic.

Rosemary helps combat the effects of water retention

Rosemary also has therapeutic properties as a mild diuretic that makes it effective in reducing swollen ankles and bloating. Dr M Halaoui from the department of Biology, University of Fez in Morocco, has studied the effects of rosemary extract's diuretic actions on the kidney.

He found that a daily dose of rosemary extract in liquid form (10 ml/Kg of weight containing 8 per cent of rosemary) can improve kidney function significantly, increase urine flow, and preserve the essential minerals sodium, potassium and chlorium (*Halaoui M et al. J Ethnopharmacol 2000; 71(3): 465-472*). This is important because conventional diuretics (water tablets) may actually worsen kidney function by speeding up the elimination of these essential minerals.

Rosemary chicken with a kick

This recipe serves 4 people

For this dish you will need the following ingredients:

4 skinless chicken breast fillets
2 tsp fresh rosemary (minced)
1 tsp sweet paprika
1 tsp sweet chilli powder
½ tsp freshly ground black pepper
½ tsp crushed coriander seeds
1 tbsp extra virgin olive oil

To prepare:

Mix the extra virgin olive oil, rosemary, paprika, chilli powder, black pepper and coriander seeds in a small bowl. Rub the spice mixture over the chicken fillets.

Cook at high heat on a heavy cast-iron griddle, in a heavy frying pan, or on a barbecue. Grill the chicken, turning once, for about five minutes – or until cooked through.

Serve immediately.

Turmeric: Helps reduce the number and severity of IBS attacks... meaning less abdominal pain and bloating

Turmeric contains an active ingredient called curcumin, a spicy yellow pigment that is used both for cooking purposes and as a medicine. Curcumin is thought to be responsible for inhibiting inflammation and tissue damage, especially in the gut, in addition to infections such as the common cold (*J Assoc Physicians India. 1998 Aug;46(8): 708-10; Food Chem Toxicol. 2000 Nov; 38(11): 991-5*).

The healing properties of turmeric (*Curcuma longa*), a perennial herb and member of the ginger plant family, have been known about by Ayurvedic (ancient Indian) practitioners for many centuries. However, it has only been recently that scientific research has begun to confirm and endorse its multiple health benefits.

Now, a new study conducted at the University of Reading has revealed yet another condition turmeric can help treat: Irritable Bowel Syndrome (IBS). Researchers found that standardised turmeric extracts can provide significant relief from the symptoms of IBS such as abdominal pain and flatulence (*Bundy R, Walker AF, Middleton RW, Booth J. Aliment Pharmacol Ther 2004*).

This is good news considering that one in five adults suffers from IBS in the UK. As well as causing abdominal pain and flatulence, as mentioned earlier, IBS can also trigger abdominal bloating, diarrhoea and/or constipation, and a sudden urgent feeling of needing the toilet straight away as soon as the pain starts.

Far from being simply an annoying condition, IBS can significantly disrupt sufferers' lives, causing a great deal of anxiety about having to go out without having immediate access to a toilet. It can also be extremely embarrassing for sufferers if they have to suddenly get up in the middle of a meeting or appointment to make an urgent dash for the toilet... leaving friends and colleagues wondering what has happened.

> *"... Turmeric extracts can play a role in improving IBS symptoms and health-related quality of life"*

The Reading University study involved 207 IBS sufferers, who were otherwise healthy. The researchers then divided the patients into two groups. The first group received a daily supplement of turmeric extract, while the second group were given two tablets of turmeric extract a day instead of one. At the end of the eight-week study the scientists found that those who were treated with one tablet a day reported a 53 per cent reduction in their symptoms, while those who were given two tablets reported a 60 per cent improvement. This included a reduction in abdominal pain, less frequent bouts of diarrhoea, and an improvement in the patients' overall quality of life.

Commenting on the findings, lead researcher Dr Rafe Bundy from the University of Reading, says: "This study shows that turmeric extracts can play a role in improving IBS symptoms and health-related quality of life in otherwise healthy adults. The results are encouraging for sufferers of this very common condition, and more extensive studies are now warranted. We may decide to experiment on the additional benefits of turmeric mixed with other natural remedies such as artichoke and St John's wort, which help improve digestion and relieve anxiety related to IBS."

It is thought that turmeric is so effective against IBS because of its well-documented anti-inflammatory action (*Curcuma longa (turmeric): Monograph. Alt Med Rev 2001, 6 Suppl: S62-66*). Inflammation plays a major role in triggering an IBS attack. Doctors believe that stress, anxiety and food intolerance, in genetically susceptible individuals, causes an inflammatory reaction within the bowel, which results in the production of toxic chemicals such as histamine, TNF-alpha and interleukin. Researchers have found that turmeric extracts are able to specifically inhibit the production of TNF-alpha and histamine during an inflammatory reaction (*Baek OS, Kang OH et al. Clin Chim Acta 2003, 338(1-2) 135-141*).

Turmeric fights inflammation and abnormal bowel muscle contractions

Another study performed at the Jack Bell Research Centre, Children and Women's Hospital in Vancouver, Canada, showed that curcumin, the active ingredient of turmeric, reduces the production of an inflammatory chemical called NF-kappa B. This chemical is involved in a variety of inflammatory conditions such as arthritis, dementia and bowel disease. The scientists discovered that turmeric is able to reduce inflammation in the lining of the bowel and improve overall bowel health (*Salh B, Assi K, Templeman V et al. Am J Physiol Gastrointest Liver Physiol 2003, 285(1): G235-243*).

Inflammation is not the only change that takes place in the bowel during an IBS attack. The small muscles around the bowel can also become irritated and cause muscle cramps, which is manifested by the sensation of needing to get to a toilet straight away. Scientists from the Department of Pharmacology, Chulalongkorn University in Bangkok, Thailand, have reported that turmeric significantly blocks these abnormal muscle cramps and relaxes the bowel muscles, so helping to improve the movements of the smooth muscle within the bowel.

As mentioned earlier, turmeric is able to block the chemical histamine, which can also cause the small muscles of the bowel to contract abnormally (*Itthipanichpong C et al. J Med Thai 2003, 2: S299-309*).

This dual action, namely turmeric's ability to reduce bowel inflammation and control abnormal muscle contractions in the bowel, translates into less frequent and less severe IBS attacks. In particular, as the functioning of the bowel becomes more normal following treatment with turmeric, less gas is produced inside the bowel, and fewer cramps and bouts of diarrhoea result.

Spicy pumpkin curry with turmeric

This recipe serves 4 people

For this dish you will need the following ingredients:

500g pumpkin, peeled and diced
1 green chilli
¼ tsp turmeric
1 tsp ginger
1 tbsp coriander seeds
1 tbsp peanut oil
¼ tsp cumin
Salt and pepper
A few coriander leaves

To prepare:

Cut the chilli in half, remove the seeds and chop. Heat the oil in a frying pan and brown the chilli. Add the diced pumpkin, turmeric, ginger and coriander seeds.

Add ½ a glass of hot water, cover and leave to cook over a low heat until the pumpkin is tender and the water has been absorbed.

Serve on a bed of brown rice and decorate with coriander leaves.

CHAPTER 6

Nuts: The snack that can benefit your health in numerous ways... from preventing heart disease to boosting immunity

Nuts are packed full of protein and are a good source of healthy fats, not to mention all the vitamins (including antioxidants) and minerals they contain. Unfortunately, many people aren't deriving any of these important health benefits, cutting nuts out of their diet because of their fatty nature and high calorie content.

Yes, nuts are high in fat but they contain high levels of healthy fats that are known to have heart-protective benefits. As Lawrence Kirk, a naturopath and lecturer in diet and medicine at the British College of Osteopathic Medicine, explains: "What many people don't appreciate is that the fat contained in nuts is mostly the healthiest monounsaturated type. Most nuts are quite low in artery-clogging saturated fats."

And Dr Hannah Theobald, a nutrition scientist for the British Nutrition Foundation in London, says: "Numerous studies have shown that replacing saturated fatty acids in the diet with unsaturated fats can lower bad, low-density lipoprotein cholesterol (LDL)." It is LDL cholesterol that increases the risk of heart disease and strokes.

The famous Nurses Health Study, which included over 86,000 participants, is an example of the heart-protective benefits of nuts. The participants in this study who ate nuts at least five times a week were found to have a 35 per cent lower risk of heart disease compared with those who rarely ate nuts or avoided them.

In addition, research conducted by Professor Penny Kris-Etherton of Pennsylvania State University, found that participants who ate peanuts and peanut butter experienced a 10 per cent reduction in triglycerides and also lowered their levels of LDL cholesterol. High triglyceride levels, like LDL cholesterol, are strongly implicated in increasing the incidence of cardiovascular disease. Better still, those involved in the trial gained these added cardiovascular benefits without gaining weight.

Eating a broad range of nuts is best as they each have specific health benefits

Another reason to eat more peanuts is because they are an excellent source of B vitamins, including folate, riboflavin and niacin. All of which are essential for healthy metabolism and growth; a deficiency of them can cause muscle degradation and fatigue.

Eating walnuts can protect your arteries... even following a high-fat meal

Spanish researchers have found that walnuts – a rich source of omega-3 alpha-linolenic acid (ALA) – can improve artery function and heart health, and may be more important in the Mediterranean diet than olive oil.

As Dr Emilio Ros, Director of the Lipid Clinic at Hospital Clínico in Barcelona, where the research was carried out, explained: "Each time we eat a high-fat meal, the fat molecules trigger an inflammatory reaction that, among other ill effects, reduces the elasticity of the arteries. Over time, this repeated damage is thought to contribute to hardening of the arteries and, in turn, to heart disease. Our latest research shows that eating walnuts helps to maintain the elasticity of the arteries."

The study investigated the effects of the addition of walnuts or olive oil to a fatty meal on a series of cardiovascular health factors. Twelve healthy people and 12 patients with high cholesterol levels were randomly assigned to a high-fat meal (80 grams fat, 35 per cent saturated fat) supplemented with 40 grams of walnuts or 25 grams of olive oil. One week later, the participants were crossed over to eat the other supplemented high-fat meal.

Following a series of tests, the researchers found that both the olive oil and the walnuts helped to decrease the sudden onset of inflammation and oxidation in the arteries, which can both lead to hardening of the arteries.

But unlike olive oil, adding walnuts also helped to preserve the elasticity and flexibility of the arteries, regardless of people's cholesterol levels. This elasticity allows the arteries to expand when needed to increase blood flow to the body (*Journal of the American College of Cardiology, published online ahead of print*).

Commenting on the findings, Dr Ros explained: "The inner lining of the arteries produces a substance called nitric oxide that is needed to keep the arteries flexible. When we eat high-fat meals, the fat molecules temporarily disrupt the production of nitric oxide, preventing the arteries from increasing blood flow in response to physical activity.

"One of the nutrients found in walnuts," he said, "is arginine, an amino acid used by the body to produce nitric oxide. Walnuts also contain antioxidants and alpha-linolenic acid (ALA), a plant-based omega-3 fatty acid. Olive oil does not contain ALA, a specific type of healthy, polyunsaturated fat."

Another must are Brazil nuts. A recent study conducted at the University of Illinois in the US, suggests that Brazil nuts may play a vital role in preventing breast cancer. According to the scientists who carried out the study, this benefit is probably a result of the high amounts of selenium they contain.

Selenium is a powerful antioxidant that helps neutralise harmful free radicals that can attack healthy cells and increase the risk of serious conditions like heart disease and cancer – including breast cancer as already mentioned, in addition to lung and bowel cancer. A deficiency of selenium is also a major factor in the development of prostate cancer.

The list of health benefits attached to each individual nut is endless. Other nuts that are particularly good, include: pistachios for their high iron, protein and fibre content and high levels of magnesium, which helps control blood pressure; hazelnuts because they are one of the richest sources of the antioxidant vitamin E; and cashew nuts for their high iron content which is needed to make haemoglobin – the red pigment in the blood.

Obviously it goes without saying that nuts should not be eaten by anyone with an allergy to them. The British Nutrition Foundation recommends that if you have a family history of nut allergies you should avoid nuts when pregnant and should not give them to your children to eat in their early years.

Broccoli and walnut salad with apple vinaigrette sauce

This recipe serves 4 people

For this dish you will need the following ingredients:

1 head of broccoli, cut into florets
3 tbsp of chopped walnuts
2 courgettes, trimmed and cut into fine matchstick strips
2 celery stalks, trimmed and cut on the diagonal
1 small bunch radishes, trimmed and quartered

For the apple vinaigrette sauce:
1 tbsp Dijon mustard
2 tbsp white miso paste
1 tsp toasted sesame oil
3 tbsp freshly pressed apple juice

To prepare:

Bring a medium-sized saucepan of water to the boil. Add the broccoli and blanch for two to three minutes. Strain and run under the cold water tap until completely cold.

Place the broccoli in a salad bowl with the courgettes, celery, walnuts and radishes.

Place the vinaigrette ingredients in a screw-top jar and shake well to blend. Pour the vinaigrette over the salad and serve.

Chunky nut and vegetable roast

This recipe serves 2 people

For this dish you will need the following ingredients:

1 carrot, chopped
1 onion, chopped
1 stick celery, chopped
200g mixed nuts (e.g. almonds, peanuts, brazil nuts) – chopped
2 tsp Marmite
2 free range eggs
2 tsp mixed herbs
Salt and pepper
Dried breadcrumbs (for coating tin)

To Prepare:

Preheat oven at 190°C/375°F/Gas Mark 5.

Put the vegetables and nuts in a bowl and mix with the remaining ingredients. Line a loaf tin with a strip of non-stick paper, grease well and sprinkle with dry breadcrumbs. Spoon mixture into tin and level the top. Bake uncovered for 45 mins until set.

CHAPTER 7

Fats: Separating the good from the bad

For years now, the low-fat pundits have been nagging us to eat less fat... claiming it is detrimental to health and can increase the risk of serious conditions like heart disease.

However, the medical profession has blamed the general consumption of fat, without distinguishing between the different kinds, for the huge rise in obesity and heart disease in the last 50 years.

While we've all had it drummed into us countless times to follow a low-fat diet, the fact remains that obesity and heart disease continue to be a major problem.

Yes, certain fats, like saturated fats found in lard and butter, can be detrimental when eaten in excess. However, others like monounsaturated fats (found in olive oil, avocados and nuts) and polyunsaturated fats (found in oily fish and hemp seed oil) are absolutely vital for good health and are needed for stamina, brain function, to build hormones and keep your skin soft and your weight down (*Udo Erasmus. Fats that Heal, Fats that Kill. Alive Books, 1993*).

A low-fat diet can seriously compromise your health

The truth is that the experts got it wrong. Worse, low-fat products are loaded with sugar that elevate blood fat levels, placing you at greater risk of high cholesterol, heart disease, stroke and Type 2 diabetes (*J. Nutrition 131:2074,2001; Am.J.Clin.Nutr. 72(5): 1128-34,2000*).

As already mentioned, certain fats are vital to your health and well-being. Healthy fats include 'monounsaturated' fats – found in olive oil, rapeseed oil, avocados, and nuts. They help lower LDL 'bad' cholesterol levels.

Including more olive oil in your diet could help lower your risk of cancer

The benefits of following a Mediterranean-style diet – rich in olive oil as well as cereals, wine, fruits, nuts, legumes, whole grains and fish – just seem to get better and better. Most of the research up until now has concentrated on the well-documented, heart-protective benefits that the diet provides.

Now a new study carried out by researchers from five different European countries has concentrated on one vital aspect of the diet – olive oil. They have found that the greater intake of olive oil in Southern European countries may be responsible for the lower rates of cancer observed among individuals living there, in comparison with their Northern European neighbours (*The Journal of the Federation of American Societies for Experimental Biology January 2007*).

The research team led by Dr Henrik E. Poulsen, of Rigshospitalet, Denmark gave volunteers from Denmark, Finland, Germany, Italy, and Spain 25 millilitres of olive oil each day for three weeks. Urine samples were then analyzed for levels of the waste by-products of cellular oxidative damage, which is a precursor of cancer. While the by-products were higher among Northern European participants at the beginning of the trial, a significant reduction was observed by the study's end.

Commenting on the findings, Dr Poulsen said: "Determining the health benefits of any particular food is challenging because it

---

involves relatively large numbers of people over significant periods of time. In our study, we overcame these challenges by measuring how olive oil affected the oxidation of our genes, which is closely linked to development of disease. This approach allows us to determine if olive oil or any other food makes a difference. Our findings must be confirmed, but every piece of evidence so far points to olive oil being a healthy food."

There are two types of 'polyunsaturated' fatty acids that you cannot function without. They are alpha-linolenic acid (LNA), an omega-3 essential fatty acid, and linoleic acid (LA), an omega-6 essential fatty acid. To make sure you're getting enough of both, take one to two tablespoons of hemp seed oil a day (keep the bottle in the fridge).

Our bodies should be able to make many other healing fatty acids from LNA and LA, but as we get older the conversion process becomes less efficient so we usually need to get at least two other omega-3 fatty acids, eicosapentaenoic acid (EPA) and docosahexaenoic acid (DHA) from our diet. These essential fatty acids are derived from dietary sources like salmon, mackerel, sardines, trout, haddock, seeds and nuts. You can also take fish oil capsules each day to ensure you're getting adequate levels of EPA and DHA.

Essential fatty acids can reduce the risk of a heart attack by 50%

Many studies have shown the benefits of essential fatty acids in preventing and treating disease. Those in fish oils have been found to lower blood pressure, prevent blood platelets from clumping and dramatically lower blood fat levels (*Am. J. Clin. Nutr. 65: 1645(S)-54(S), 1997; Am. J. Clin. Nutr. 72: 389-94, 2000*).

In fact, one major study has calculated that just eating more salmon and cold-water fish can cut the risk of a fatal heart attack by up to 50 per cent (*J. Amer. Med. Assoc. 274: 1363-7, 1995*). Fish oils and flaxseed oil have been linked with a significantly lower incidence of breast cancer (*Nutr. Cancer 24: 151-60, 1995*), and have been found to prevent changes in the cells lining the large intestine that can lead to colon cancer (*Nutr. Rev. 8(51): 241-3, 1994*).

These same oils can suppress the self-destructive process of rheumatoid arthritis, in which the immune system attacks healthy joint tissue (*Prostaglandins, Leukotrienes Ess. Fatty Acids 56: 193-8, 1997*). Evening primrose oil and borage oil can also reduce morning stiffness, joint swelling and tenderness and increase joint mobility in people with rheumatoid and osteoarthritis (*Arth. Rheum. 33: 1526-32, 1990; Arth. Rheum. 39: 1808-17, 1996*).

How we've been duped over 'healthy' oils for cooking

However, there is one drawback with polyunsaturated fatty acids – they quickly become oxidised when exposed to light and heat. In this state, they lose their beneficial properties and produce toxins and free radicals that can damage your body's cells.

So, always keep oils in a cool, dark cupboard or in your fridge and never use polyunsaturated oils such as rapeseed or sunflower seed oils for deep-frying. Food manufacturers persuaded us years ago to change from 'dangerous' fats like lard and butter to 'healthy' polyunsaturated oils – but they forgot to tell us that these oils are the worst choice you can make for cooking foods.

Butter is definitely a better alternative for frying foods than polyunsaturated oils. Your best choice is to opt for extra virgin olive oil – an unrefined oil that keeps its chemical structure well when heated and doesn't produce as many free radicals. But frying at high temperatures for long periods causes any fat, and the food fried in it, to break down and produce toxic and cancer-causing chemicals. Quick stir-frying is much healthier.

In addition, steer clear of trans-fatty acids, which are found in margarine and other processed foods. They have been found to impair the functioning of the immune system, reduce liver function, and reduce testosterone production (*Udo Erasmus. Fats that Heal, Fats that Kill. Alive Books, 1993*). They are created in the laboratory when food industry manufacturers add hydrogen to unsaturated vegetable oil, in a process known as hydrogenation, which turns them into harmful saturated fats.

Virgin coconut oil: The unique saturated fat that actually promotes weight loss

There is one saturated fat that, unlike the majority, can actually help maintain good health and promote weight loss. Its name is virgin coconut oil. Traditionally used in tropical regions for centuries, researchers have noted that the Polynesians and the Bicolanos of the Philippines, who include virgin coconut oil in their diets each day, have normal cholesterol levels and little incidence of coronary disease (*Bartimeus P. Facing Fats: vegetable oils unbottled. Optimum Nutrition journal 2003; 16(3): 38-43*).

In fact, amongst these populations, digestive problems are rare, as are other problems including colitis, colon cancer, kidney stones, underactive thyroid and obesity.

So what makes virgin coconut oil different from most saturated fats?

There are three main groups of saturated fats: short chain, medium chain and long chain. Each type has different nutritional and biological characteristics. For example, long chain fatty acids (LCFA) – present in foods such as beef, mutton, pork and dairy products – cause blood platelets to become sticky, which can lead to cardiovascular disease and related conditions.

However, medium chain fatty acids (MCFA), as found in virgin coconut oil, do not act in the same way. These fatty acids are of smaller particle size, making them more water-soluble and therefore easier to digest. They are also metabolised quickly and used as a source of energy rather than being converted to and stored as fat.

Virgin coconut oil contains several types of MCFAs: lauric acid, myristic acid, caprylic acid and capric acid. Lauric acid makes up about 50 per cent of the fatty acid content in coconut oil; the only other abundant source in nature is found in human breast milk.

According to Dr Mary Enig, a nutritionist and biochemist and one of the world's leading authorities on fats and oils: "Lauric acid is a medium chain fatty acid, which has the additional beneficial function of being formed into monolaurin in the human or animal body. Monolaurin is the antiviral, antibacterial, and antiprotozoal monoglyceride used by the human or animal to destroy viruses such as HIV, herpes, influenza, various pathogenic bacteria including Listeria monocytogenes [which can cause septicaemia, meningitis and encephalitis] and Helicobacter pylori [implicated in stomach ulcers], and protozoa such as Giardia lamblia [which can cause diarrhoea and stomach cramps." (*Dr Mary Enig, Know Your Fats: The Complete Primer for Understanding the Nutrition of Fats, Oils and Cholesterol, Bethesda Press, 2000*).

Virgin coconut oil kick-starts your metabolism – helping you to burn fat fast

One of the interesting things about virgin coconut oil is that it contains fewer calories than most other fats. Generally, fats contain 9 calories per gram, but Dr Bruce Fife, author of *The Healing Miracles of Coconut Oil*, states that MCFAs contain only 6.8 calories per gram. So by replacing other fats with coconut oil you'll be getting fewer calories.

In addition, because virgin coconut oil is utilised in a different way to other fats, it can actually aid weight loss (as part of a calorie controlled diet), rather than discourage it. This is because normally when a fat is digested, the resulting fatty acids enter the bloodstream and are then deposited into fat cells. However, the MCFAs in virgin coconut oil do not enter your bloodstream but go straight to your liver where they are immediately converted to energy. Only when an excess of the oil is eaten is it converted to fat.

Another factor that gives coconut oil the thumbs up to dieters, is that it helps increase your metabolic rate. MCFAs appear to shift the metabolism into a higher gear, enabling your body to burn more calories.

In one study, the thermogenic (fat-burning) effect of a high calorie diet containing 40 per cent fat as MCFAs and 40 per cent fat as LCFAs was compared. The results showed that the fat-burning effect of the MCFA diet was almost twice as great (*Hill JO, et al. Thermogenesis in man during overfeeding with medium chain triglycerides. Metabolism 1990; 38: 641-8*). In another study, researchers compared meals consisting of 400 calories made up of either entirely MCFAs or LCFAs. The fat burning effect of the MCFA meal was three times as high than the LCFA meal, over a six-hour period (*Seaton TB, et al. Thermic effect of medium-chain and long-chain triglycerides in man. Am. J. of Clin. Nutr. 1986; 44: 630*).

How to benefit your health

The recommended dosage for virgin coconut oil is one tablespoon a day. It's important that you only purchase 'virgin' coconut oil, as this means it's unrefined and has been extracted with minimal heat to ensure that its active constituents remain intact. Many supermarkets only sell refined coconut oil, which is very unhealthy. Refined oils are extracted at high temperatures and chemical solvents are used to pull the oil from the seed or nut. In addition, most of the active beneficial constituents are destroyed during this process.

Virgin coconut oil can be used as a healthy replacement to cooking oils for sautéing and stir-frying. Other ways of adding it to your diet include blending it into shakes or smoothies, stirring it into porridge, or using it to roast vegetables.

Because of its high saturated fatty acid content, virgin coconut oil is naturally solid at room temperature or when kept in the fridge, which makes it ideal as a substitute for butter or margarine. It can be used for spreading or for baking and has a light coconut flavour. The oil will start to become liquid at temperatures in excess of 18°C. Due to its solidity at room temperature it is not suitable as a salad dressing.

Virgin coconut oil can also be used externally and applied neat to the skin. It is said to sooth sunburn and may help improve conditions such as psoriasis and eczema when applied to the affected area.

There are no contraindications associated with virgin coconut oil, and it has a shelf life of 18 months.

Sautéed sea bass with virgin coconut oil and garlic

This recipe serves 2 people

For this dish you will need the following ingredients:

450g of sea bass fillets
1 tbsp of virgin coconut oil
4 cloves of garlic (chopped)
½ a red onion (thinly chopped)
2 tbsp of fresh coriander
The juice of one large lemon

To prepare:

Melt the virgin coconut oil on a teppenyaki grill or heavy frying pan. Add the fish and sauté for five minutes, turning over only once. Remove the fish from the pan and pour in all the other ingredients, allowing them to heat through. This takes approximately a minute and a half, then pour these other ingredients over the fish and serve immediately.

Roasted vegetables in extra virgin olive oil with couscous

This recipe serves 4 people

For this dish you will need the following ingredients:

7 tbsp of extra virgin olive oil
2 tbsp of harissa sauce (available at most supermarkets)
1 red pepper (deseeded and quartered)
1 orange pepper (deseeded and quartered)
1 aubergine (sliced into batons)
2 red onions (cut into wedges)
4 large chillies (halved)
Salt and pepper
125g couscous
Bunch of fresh parsley (chopped)
Juice of half a lemon

To prepare:

Preheat your oven to 190C/375F/Gas Mark 5. Place all the vegetables in a large roasting tray and drizzle with four tablespoons of olive oil and season with the salt and pepper. Toss the vegetables in the tray to make sure they are coated, then place in the oven and roast for 25 minutes turning regularly. Put the couscous in a bowl and pour 200ml of boiling water over it. Leave to stand for five minutes until the couscous has absorbed all the water. Mix together the remaining olive oil, parsley, lemon juice and harissa sauce. Divide the couscous between four bowls and then add the roasted vegetables on top, along with the harissa sauce. Serve immediately.

CHAPTER 8

Fish has proven protective benefits for many of your body's most important organs

In the previous chapter on 'good and bad' fats, you discovered that one of the best dietary source of omega-3 fatty acids is fish, especially dark-meat fish like swordfish and tuna. And while a high intake of these deep-water fish presents the potential problem of ingesting too much mercury, the importance of omega-3 to our overall health (and heart health in particular) can't be emphasised enough.

A study carried out at the University of Washington in the US has shown that how you prepare your fish also makes a difference. The study examined the diets of almost 4,000 adults over the age of 65 who showed no signs of cardiovascular disease. Researchers followed up nine years later to record the subjects' incidence of non-fatal heart attacks, and deaths due to the narrowing of arteries that causes coronary heart disease (CHD).

The study results showed that those who regularly ate tuna and other baked or broiled fish (three or more times per week) had a significantly lower risk of CHD than those who ate the same fish infrequently. Those who regularly ate fried fish, however, had a higher risk of both heart attack and death due to CHD (*Journal of the American Heart Association, 2003 Mar 18; 107(10); 1372-7*).

Eating fish as little as once a week could lower your risk of Alzheimer's by up to 60%

Oily fish – including, salmon, mackerel, tuna, herring and sardines – has also been shown to help ward off age-related memory loss and even lower the risk of Alzheimer's disease.

A seven-year US study, involved 815 participants in the Chicago Health and Aging project, who were aged 65 and older. Follow-up evaluation tests nearly four years later found that 131 participants had developed Alzheimer's.

The researchers found that those participants who ate fish (including tuna, shellfish and fish sticks) once a week had a 60 per cent lower risk of developing the disease, than those who never or rarely ate fish. The researchers came to this conclusion after taking into account and making adjustments for other possible risk factors, including age, sex, ethnicity and associated conditions like heart disease.

As already mentioned oily fish is one of the richest sources of omega-3 – thought to be important for brain development. However, this study found that these benefits were not limited to fish alone, but also applied to those participants who derived omega-3 fatty acids from other dietary sources, such as dark green leafy vegetables and nuts.

Although more studies are needed, this research adds to the mounting body of evidence regarding the health-related benefits linked to omega-3 fatty acids. It also supports the results of previous animal studies, which have revealed how animals fed omega-3 fatty acids showed improved learning abilities and memory.

Age-related macular degeneration – how omega-3 fatty acids hold the key to healthy eyes

Recent research findings have also revealed how a high intake of omega-3 fatty acids and oily fish may offer vital protection against advanced cases of age-related macular degeneration (ARMD) (*American Medical Association journal Archives of Ophthalmology May 2007*).

ARMD is currently the leading cause of vision loss in people over 55, and by the age of 65 it's estimated that as many as one in four of us in the UK may begin to show signs of having the condition.

The disease involves progressive damage to the central and most vital area of your retina – the light-sensitive tissue at the back of your eye. This area is called the macula, from the latin word for spot. It's what allows you to focus on objects directly in front of you, which is essential for seeing fine detail and is needed for activities like reading and driving. Sufferers often experience shape distortion, have difficulty seeing objects far away, close objects can appear blurred and, in more advanced cases, a dark patch can appear in the centre of their field of vision.

The study, conducted by researchers at The Age-Related Eye Disease Study Research Group, involved 4,519 individuals aged between 60 and 80 upon enrolment. The participants completed questionnaires concerning their previous year's dietary intake, and underwent retinal photography to assess the presence and stage of macular degeneration.

While 1,115 participants were free of ARMD symptoms, 2,746 were classified in intermediate stages, and 658 were found to have advanced (neovascular) age-related macular degeneration. The research team determined that a greater intake of omega-3 fatty acids, including oily fish, was associated with a reduced risk of advanced disease. When oily fish intake was examined, consuming more than two servings per week appeared to provide the greatest protection.

Commenting on the findings the researchers said: "Dietary total omega-3 long-chain polyunsaturated fatty acid intake was inversely associated with neovascular ARMD, as was docosahexaenoic acid. Higher fish consumption, both total and broiled/baked, was also inversely associated with neovascular ARMD."

Omega-3 fatty acids docosahexaenoic acid and eicosapentaenoic acid may protect the retina by influencing gene expression, retinal cell differentiation, and survival. Other properties of the fatty acids may also be involved, including their ability to reduce inflammation.

On the subject of seafood, oysters are a healthy choice. Six oysters pack an amazing 500 per cent of your RDA for zinc – vital for building a healthy immune system, as well as repairing and maintaining muscle tissue. Many runners are more susceptible to viral and bacterial infections after competitive events such as a marathon, and research shows that zinc can protect them against these consequences (*Appl Environ Microbiol. 1999 Jul; 65(7): 3015-20*). Zinc is essential for sperm production, and for sexual functioning in both men and women.

This spicy mackerel dish provides a tasty way to top up your levels of omega-3

This recipe serves 4 people

For this dish you will need the following ingredients:

4 large fresh mackerel (gutted)
2 medium aubergines (diced)
3 tbsp extra virgin olive oil
3 garlic cloves

1 small bunch of fresh coriander
1 red chilli (deseeded)
1 medium onion (thinly sliced)
400g can plum tomatoes
1 tsp sweet paprika
½ tsp ground cumin
Pinch of saffron strands
2 heaped tbsp full-fat Greek natural yoghurt
Sea salt
Lemon wedges, to serve (optional)

To prepare:

Preheat the oven to 200C/400F/Gas Mark 6.

Season the mackerel with coarsely ground sea salt and set aside.

Place the aubergine in a large roasting tin, drizzle with two tablespoons of the extra virgin olive oil. Cook for 20-25 minutes in the oven, tossing halfway, or until just tender. Remove and set aside. Increase the oven temperature to 240C/475F/Gas Mark 9.

Meanwhile, separate the coriander leaves from the stalks or roots and set the leaves aside in a cool place. Chop the stalks or roots with the chilli and crushed garlic until it's almost a paste. Heat the remaining oil in a frying pan over a low heat. Cook the coriander paste and onion for 10 minutes, stirring occasionally.

Drain the canned tomatoes in a colander and get rid of any excess juices. Add the canned tomatoes to the pan with the paprika, cumin, saffron and 200ml water and simmer for 20 minutes, stirring occasionally. Carefully stir in the aubergine, add a good splash of water to loosen the mixture and cook for a further 10 minutes.

Meanwhile, make two or three diagonal slashes on one side of each mackerel. Place on a baking tray lined with non-stick baking paper and bake for 10-12 minutes. Check to see that they are cooked by seeing if the flesh can be pushed off the bone with the back of a fork. When it can, remove from the oven and set aside for five minutes.

Take the pan of spiced aubergines off the heat. Roughly chop the reserved coriander leaves and stir most of them into the aubergines, along with the yoghurt. Season to taste and spoon onto four warm plates. Carefully lift the fish on top of the aubergines and scatter with the remaining chopped coriander. Serve with lemon wedges.

Salmon with a tangy, mango salsa twist

This dish serves 2 people

To make this dish you will need the following ingredients:

2 salmon steaks (each 250g)
1 medium red onion (finely sliced)
1 large green mango
1 cm fresh ginger root (peeled, finely sliced, and chopped)
1 large green chilli (deseeded and finely sliced)
1 tbsp green peppercorns
The juice of 4 limes
2 tbsp extra virgin olive oil (for mixing and brushing)
1 pinch salt
1 pinch sugar
4 basil leaves
1 bunch coriander
2 sprigs mint

To prepare:

To prepare the salsa, soak the finely sliced red onion in ice water for five minutes, then drain.

Peel the green mango, then slice the flesh with a potato peeler and set aside. Mix together the sliced mango, chilli, ginger, green peppercorns, juice of three limes and red onion. Add olive oil to taste, plus salt and a pinch of sugar. Set aside.

Preheat a griddle pan until extremely hot. Season the salmon with salt and the remaining lime juice. Brush with olive oil. Cook the salmon on the griddle for two to three minutes on each side.

Meanwhile, roughly chop the basil, coriander and mint and add to the mango salsa.

Serve the freshly griddled salmon with the green mango salsa.

Grilled oysters in lemon butter

This recipe serves 4 people

For this dish you will need the following ingredients:

24 oysters
6 cloves garlic
2 tbsp chopped tarragon
1 shallot, finely diced
1 tbsp parsley
250g butter
1 lemon, zest grated and juiced
100g parmesan, grated
2kg coarse sea salt

To prepare:

Preheat your oven to 230C/450F/Gas Mark 8.

Soften the butter. Mix with all of the ingredients except the oysters and parmesan. Set in the fridge. Open the oysters and drain all of the liquid from them. Place on to a tray of sea salt, ensuring all oysters are securely flat. Put a one centimetre square chunk of butter on to each oyster, followed by a sprinkle of parmesan. Bake in the oven for five minutes. Serve with brown bread and lemon.

Monkfish and veggie mix

This recipe serves 5 people

For this dish you will need the following ingredients:

550g of monkfish (skinned and cubed)
2 tbsp of extra virgin olive oil
1 red pepper (seeded and chopped)
1 small onion (finely chopped)
115g mushrooms (finely sliced)
1 green courgette (sliced)
400g canned chopped tomatoes
3 cloves of garlic (crushed or finely chopped)
1 tbsp of tomato purée
½ tsp of dried oregano
2 tbsp fresh parsley (chopped)
150ml of dry red wine
Salt and pepper
6-8 fresh basil leaves (shredded) to garnish

To prepare:

Heat the oil in a large saucepan over a medium heat. Add the pepper, onion and mushrooms and cook for five minutes. Add the garlic, parsley, oregano and tomato purée and stir well. Pour in the wine and tomatoes and stir. Season with salt and pepper and bring the mixture to the boil. Then simmer gently for 15 minutes. Add the courgette slices and monkfish. Cover and simmer for a further 15 minutes or until the monkfish is cooked. Sprinkle with basil and serve immediately.

Salad niçoise

This recipe serves 4 people

For this dish you will need the following ingredients:

6 or 8 lettuce leaves from the heart of a crisp iceberg lettuce
3 hard boiled eggs (cut into quarters)
14 new baby potatoes (halved lengthways)
6 medium-sized tomatoes (cut into quarters)
500g can of tuna
6 anchovy fillets
16 black olives
4 tablespoons of extra virgin olive oil
1 tbsp of wine vinegar
2 tbsp of chopped fresh parsley
1 clove of garlic (crushed)
1 tsp of capers
Salt and pepper

To prepare:

Cook the new potatoes in a pan of water for 10-15 minutes, or until the potatoes are just tender. Drain and leave to cool.

Place the lettuce leaves, tomatoes, eggs and potatoes in a salad bowl. Roughly flake the tuna over this mixture.

Pour the olive oil and vinegar into a screw top jar and add the garlic, capers and parsley. Shake well. Pour over the salad and toss lightly. Scatter the olives over the salad and lay the anchovy fillets on top.

CHAPTER 9

Meat helps provide your body with fuel

If you eat meat, it is a good idea to purchase organic meat only. Yes, it may cost more but the extra expense is definitely worth it in terms of your health. More information on this is given under the 'Is organic food really better?' section on page 201, but to summarise it means that you are not consuming meat that has been treated with growth and sex hormones or antibiotics.

Meat should be eaten in moderation in order to ensure you're not getting too many saturated fats or acid in your diet.

Meats are harder to digest and absorb than foods of vegetable origin. However, poultry is far easier to digest than red meat. Plus, if you remove the skin then the meat's fat content is considerably reduced, as most of the fat is located just under the skin.

Turkey is an excellent protein choice as it is incredibly low in fat and nutrient rich. It contains zinc, niacin, selenium, and vitamins B6 and B12 that can help lower your risk of heart disease and cancer. It's a great choice if you suffer from insomnia too, as it contains large amounts of tryptophan, which is a natural sleeping aid. Plus it is relatively inexpensive compared to many other meats.

If you do like red meat then lamb, game and rabbit are good alternatives to beef or pork, as they are easier to digest than the latter. Generally, game tends to be higher in iron than other meats.

Liver and kidney are a good source of many vitamins and minerals and are low in fat.

Meat products that are made up from the wastes of other meats like sausages and burgers should definitely be avoided at all costs. Leftover flesh from animals such as lips and ears is often ground up and used in the production of sausages, burgers, frankfurters, pies and faggots. In addition, to make these products more desirable, a wide range of additives are normally added, which are completely unnatural and can cause toxins to accumulate.

Warming turkey chilli

This recipe serves 4 people

For this dish you will need the following ingredients:

500g of turkey mince
450g of new potatoes (cut into chunks)
400g can of red kidney beans
400g can of chopped tomatoes
2 tbsp of tomato purée
1 tbsp of extra virgin olive oil
1 pint of vegetable stock
1 onion (chopped)
1 red pepper (seeded and cut into chunks)
150g of baby spinach leaves
2 garlic cloves (crushed)
2 tsp chilli powder
Salt and pepper

To prepare:

Heat the oil in a large pan and fry the onion and minced turkey for five minutes, or until the onion is softened. Stir in the garlic, chilli powder, tomato purée, tomatoes, stock, red pepper, new potatoes and kidney beans. Bring to the boil, then cover and simmer for 20 minutes (until the potatoes are tender).

Stir in the spinach leaves until just wilted and season to taste.

Chicken caesar salad

This dish serves 4 people

For this dish you will need the following ingredients:

2 large cooked chicken breasts (thinly sliced)
2 tbsp of extra virgin olive oil
1 garlic clove (crushed)
1 large cos lettuce
4 tbsp of half-fat crème fraiche
2 thick slices of granary bread (crusts removed, cut into cubes)
1 tsp cajun seasoning
1 tbsp lemon juice
2 tsp Worcestershire sauce
1 tsp Dijon mustard
Parmesan cheese
Salt and pepper

To prepare:

Preheat the oven to 220C/425F/Gas Mark 7. Mix the bread cubes with one tablespoon of olive oil, the garlic and cajun seasoning. Spread on to a baking sheet and bake in the oven for eight minutes, until crisp and golden.

Tear the lettuce into pieces and toss with the spicy croutons.

Mix together the remaining olive oil, lemon juice, crème fraiche, Worcestershire sauce and Dijon mustard and season to taste.

Drizzle the mixture over the lettuce and arrange the chicken slices on top. Grate a little parmesan over the salad and serve.

Pork and spinach sesame seed stir-fry

This recipe serves 1 person

For this dish you will need the following ingredients:

4 ounces of pork loin cut into thick strips
5 ounces of fresh spinach
1 tbsp of white sesame seeds
1 clove of crushed garlic
1 tbsp of extra virgin olive oil
2 ½ ounces of spring onion sliced
¼ tsp of cayenne pepper
1 tbsp of soy sauce
1 tbsp of sesame oil

To prepare:

Toast the sesame seeds in a dry large frying pan or wok over a high heat for one to two minutes until golden brown. Remove from the pan and set aside. Heat the olive oil in a large frying pan or wok and then add the pork strips, garlic, onion, spring onion strips and cayenne pepper – stir-fry over a high heat until cooked through. Remove from the pan and set aside. Add the soy sauce and spinach to the pan and toss lightly, then cover and cook for approximately two minutes until the spinach is soft. Return the pork mixture to the pan and add the sesame seeds and sesame oil – toss well and serve immediately.

CHAPTER 10

Dairy products: uncovering common myths, particularly when it comes to milk

Raw fresh milk is very difficult to obtain as almost all milk available to us is now pasteurised. Pasteurised milk involves heating the milk in order to kill the majority of bacteria, such as bovine *tubercle bacilli* (TB), that may have been present in the milk. However this process also destroys the beneficial bacteria *Lactobacillus* that is good for the bowel and gut and helps keep the number of undesirable bacteria under control. In addition, the pasteurisation process kills many natural enzymes that aid digestion.

It can also lead to poor digestion due to the fact that it produces excessive and undesirable mucus in the intestines, which can coat the wall of the intestines and prevent the proper absorption of minerals and other nutrients.

The pasteurisation process is also unable to destroy the hormones present in milk, which cows naturally secrete. For example, human growth hormone is present in cow's milk which helps the calf grow to a full-sized cow. These hormones are very likely to have an adverse effect on humans consuming the milk.

Ironically, many people drink milk because of its high calcium content, particularly to try and help ward of osteoporosis. However, the calcium in milk is prone to poor absorption especially because of its high magnesium to calcium ratio – magnesium is essential for regulating calcium metabolism.

You can easily increase your calcium intake through other food sources such as leafy green vegetables, soya products (soya milk is a good alternative to milk providing you opt for a product that does not contain added sugar or salt), dried figs and seeds like pumpkin, sesame and sunflower seeds. In addition, many people are unable to tolerate the lactose (sugar) present in milk, which can cause abdominal bloating, gas, cramps and diarrhoea.

Milk is also linked to being a factor in causing numerous conditions including ulcerative colitis, Crohn's disease, hardening of the arteries, allergies, asthma, sinus problems, catarrh, kidney problems and even cancer.

The main advantage of skimmed milk is that it contains less saturated animal fat, which makes it a better choice in terms of reducing the risk of coronary heart disease and for weight reduction.

Cut your blood pressure in half by eating low-fat dairy

In the UK, about half of people over 65, and about one in four middle-aged adults, have high blood pressure. It is more common in people who have a family history of high blood pressure, are overweight, eat a lot of salt, don't eat enough fruits and vegetables, don't exercise, or drink a lot of alcohol.

But, new research has found that middle-aged adults who favour skimmed milk and other low-fat dairy foods may have lower blood pressure (*Am J Clin Nutr 2005; 82(5): 972-9*).

Spanish researchers examined 5,880 adults between the ages of 20 and 90 and who were free of high blood pressure and cardiovascular disease. The volunteers were asked to fill out questionnaires about their diet and other lifestyle factors.

Then after two years, they repeated the questionnaire and the researchers ran tests to find out how many had developed high blood

---

pressure. Overall, 180 people developed the condition during the study period. Those who had reported the highest intake of low-fat dairy – mostly in the form of skimmed and reduced-fat milk – were 54 per cent less likely to develop high blood pressure than those with the lowest intakes.

Even better, these benefits were after the researchers accounted for overall diet, exercise, body weight and smoking.

This study is the first to link low-fat dairy intake to lower blood pressure in middle-aged patients. Previously, research had only found benefits in children and young adults.

The findings from these studies do not prove that low-fat dairy foods have a direct benefit on blood pressure, explained Dr. Alvaro Alonso, lead researcher. But he said it at least seems that people who want to prevent high blood pressure can include low-fat dairy foods in their diets.

Milk, the researchers noted, provides certain proteins – caseins and whey proteins – that may act in a manner similar to blood pressure-lowering drugs called angiotensin converting enzyme, or ACE, inhibitors. They speculate that these proteins may help explain the study results.

So, if you are struggling to control your blood pressure, this study suggests that you may want to switch to low-fat dairy products. As always, you should consult your doctor before making any changes to your medication or diet.

There are many alternatives to cow's milk. As well as soya milk, as mentioned earlier, organic goat's milk is a good choice as it is far easier to digest than cow's milk. Rice and oat milk are also good options.

Cheese is a milk concentrate so has all the health disadvantages of milk outlined above. In addition, it is often high in sodium and should only be eaten in moderation. Goat's cheese is a better choice.

Live yoghurt has numerous health advantages. A recent study from the University of California at Davis found that people who ate two cups of yoghurt daily – the kind made with live bacteria cultures (specifically *Lactobacillus* and *Streptococcus thermophilus*) – suffered from fewer colds (*Am J Clin Nutr. 2001 Feb; 73 (2 Suppl): 444S-450S*). Also, those with allergies experienced fewer symptoms. This is thought to be due to 'friendly' bacteria in the yoghurt which help boost the immune system.

Live yoghurt is also particularly beneficial for maintaining intestinal health and helps speed up recovery from diarrhoea, gastroenteritis and candida. The beneficial bacteria cultures in live yoghurt helps restore levels of 'friendly' bacteria that become depleted following a course of antibiotics.

Yoghurt is extremely versatile and makes an excellent breakfast food when mixed with fruit, seeds and cereals. It can also be used to thicken soups, stews and sauces – however, it should not be used during cooking but simply stirred in at the end as heating destroys friendly bacteria.

Men – Lower your risk of the 3rd most common cancer by eating more calcium and dairy

According to the NHS, colorectal cancer (also called bowel cancer) is the third most common cancer in men in the UK. Each year, there are about 18,500 new cases of bowel cancer in men which can occur anywhere in the colon or rectum.

Recently, researchers from the Karolinska Institute in Stockholm,

---

Sweden found that men whose diets were high in calcium and dairy had a lower risk of developing this common cancer (*Am J Clin Nutr 2006; 83(3): 667-73*).

In 1997, the scientists enrolled 45,306 men who had no history of cancer and were between the ages of 45 to 79. They kept track of these volunteers for an average of 6.7 years. The men completed food frequency questionnaires at the beginning of the study and these were analysed by the researchers for calcium and dairy intake.

During the study 276 volunteers were diagnosed with colon cancer and 173 with rectal cancer. The researchers found that the men whose calcium intake was in the top one-fourth of all the volunteers had a 32 per cent lower risk of developing colorectal cancer. For dairy foods, consuming seven or more servings a day reduced the risk to 54 per cent when compared to the men who ate less than two servings a day.

This study suggests that dairy has the greatest protective effect on the colon. Commenting on the findings, the researchers said: "Future studies should examine the relation of other components of dairy foods, such as conjugated linoleic acid, sphingolipids and milk proteins, with the risk of colorectal cancer."

So if you want to lower your risk of developing colorectal cancer, it may be worth making sure you get enough calcium, specifically from yoghurt and cheese. If you are looking to incorporate some non-dairy food sources of calcium, you can try some of these foods: green, leafy vegetables – including broccoli, collard greens, kale, mustard greens, turnip greens and pak choi or Chinese cabbage – canned salmon and sardines, shellfish, almonds, Brazil nuts and dried beans.

Grilled salmon fillets with a herb yoghurt sauce

This recipe serves 2 people

For this dish you will need the following ingredients:

2 salmon fillets
Generous portion of broccoli
Extra virgin olive oil
Sea salt and pepper
3 tbsp plain live yoghurt
1 tbsp fresh parsley, chopped
Juice of half a lemon

To Prepare:

In a bowl add the yoghurt, the chopped herbs and lemon juice. Mix well and add sea salt to taste. Put to one side.

Brush both salmon fillets with olive oil and season. Heat the grill to a high heat, for best results use a ridged or flat griddle pan.

Meanwhile, steam the broccoli.

Place the salmon fillets skin side down on the grill pan, turn the heat down to a moderate high and cook for around four minutes before turning and cook for a further minute. Make sure the salmon is completely cooked through before serving.

Serve with the steamed broccoli and generous dollops of the herb yoghurt sauce.

Pepper, lentil and goat's cheese surprise

This recipe serves 4 people

For this dish you will need the following ingredients:

225g split red lentils
4 red peppers
2 onions, peeled
175g celery
40g butter
170g fresh soft goat's cheese
10 black olives, halved and pitted
basil sprigs, to garnish
salt and pepper

To Prepare:

Cook the lentils in boiling salted water for 12 minutes until tender and then drain.

Meanwhile, halve the peppers length-wise and remove the core and seeds. Grill the pepper halves for 10 minutes, turning occasionally, until the skin is browned and the flesh softened.

Finely chop the onions and celery. Melt the butter in a saucepan and sauté the onions and celery for two minutes. Stir in the lentils.

Spoon the filling evenly in to the pepper halves. Grill under moderate heat for two minutes until the filling is golden.

Garnish with basil sprigs and serve hot.

CHAPTER 11

Eggs – Don't let anyone try and tell you they're bad for your heart!

For a long time eggs received a bad press and many doctors were convinced that regular consumption of them increased the risk of heart disease, as they contain cholesterol. Yet research has shown that this certainly isn't the case... quite the opposite in fact, as they're now proving something of a super food.

Using the Nurse's Health Study and the Health Professionals' Follow-up Study, researcher Dr Frank Hu and his team from the Harvard School of Public Health noted that – after adjusting for age, smoking and other risk factors – there was no evidence of an association between eating whole eggs and the risk of heart disease or stroke in men or women (*JAMA 1999; 281 (15): 1387-94*).

In addition, eggs have been found to help raise levels of HDL (good) cholesterol – needed to help insulate nerve fibres, maintain cell walls, produce vitamin D and manufacture various hormones and digestive juices.

While most people know that eggs are an excellent source of protein – containing no less than eight essential amino acids (which are the building blocks of protein) – not everyone is aware that they are also packed full of vitamins and minerals. For example, they contain vitamins B12 and B6 and folic acid that help lower homocysteine levels – this is important as high levels are associated with heart disease, stroke and Alzheimer's.

As if all this wasn't reason enough for including more eggs in your diet, they also contain zinc which is essential for supporting your immune system; carotenes which offer vital protection against age-related macular degeneration; sulphur which possesses anti-inflammatory properties and antioxidant protection; and magnesium which helps fight everything from high blood pressure, migraines and atherogenesis (fatty deposits on arterial walls) (*Pathobiology 1999; 67(4): 207-13*).

Add to this mix vitamins A, D, E and K, iron, riboflavin, niacin, potassium and lipoproteins, and it's not difficult to figure out why eggs are such a nutritious and healthy food.

Asparagus and sautéed mushroom-filled omelette

This recipe serves 2 people

For this dish you will need the following ingredients:

½ lb of asparagus (chopped)
2 tbsp butter
1 garlic clove (crushed)
1 small red onion
3 cups of sliced mushrooms
4 eggs
2 tbsp milk
½ tsp salt
¼ tsp crushed dried basil
⅛ tsp freshly-ground black pepper

To prepare:

Cut the asparagus into 1-inch pieces and cook in boiling water until tender (two to four minutes); drain thoroughly.

Melt half of the butter in a medium sized frying pan over medium-high heat. Sauté the garlic, onion and mushrooms until soft (about three minutes). Remove from pan and mix with asparagus; cover and set aside to keep warm.

In a small bowl, combine the eggs, milk, salt, basil and pepper. Melt the remaining butter in the frying pan over a moderate heat and pour in the egg mixture. Tip the pan to coat evenly with egg.

As the eggs cook, periodically tilt the frying pan, lifting cooked portion, allowing uncooked egg mixture to slide beneath. When eggs are cooked, but surface is still shiny, place asparagus and mushrooms on one side; slide out of pan onto a warm plate. Fold plain half of omelette over asparagus-mushroom mixture. Serve immediately.

Eggs Florentine and haddock

This recipe serves 4

For this dish you will need the following ingredients:

225g bag young spinach leaves
50g butter
4 tomatoes, sliced
4 x 175g (6oz) smoked haddock fillets
2 tbsp plain flour
300ml (½ pint) milk
50g (1 ¾oz) Cheddar cheese, grated
4 large eggs
salt and freshly ground black pepper

To prepare:

Preheat the oven to 180C/350F/Gas Mark 4.
Empty the spinach into a large pan, cover and cook for two to three minutes or until wilted. Drain well in a sieve, pressing down with a wooden spoon to remove the excess juices. Add 15g butter and season to taste. Arrange four heaps of spinach in a shallow ovenproof dish.

Top with sliced tomatoes, then the haddock fillets on top of the spinach. Cover with buttered foil and bake for 15-20 minutes or until the fish flakes easily.

Meanwhile, place the remaining butter, flour and milk, in a medium pan and bring to the boil, whisking all the time, until the mixture boils and thickens. Cook for one minute and then remove from the heat. Stir in half the cheese and set aside.

Preheat the grill. Top each fillet with a poached egg, pour over the sauce and top with the remaining cheese. Cook for two minutes under a hot grill until golden brown.

CHAPTER 12

Honey – Discover the incredible healing honey that is showing potential against deadly hospital super bugs like MRSA

Honey is a complex mixture of sugars obtained by bees from plant nectar, combined with secretions added by the bees. This mixture is stored in the honeycomb to ripen and mature.

The sugars it contains are mainly in the form of glucose and fructose but honey is also rich in minerals, including important trace elements, and many amino acids and vitamins – including numerous B vitamins and vitamin C. The enzymes amylase, invertase and glucose oxidase are also present – the latter being responsible for honey's antibacterial activity which generates an antiseptic called hydrogen peroxide.

One honey in particular stands head and shoulders above the rest for its incredible healing powers. Manuka honey has been found to be effective against deadly infections like MRSA – the well-documented super bug which is unresponsive to antibiotics and other forms of topical treatment.

It's also beneficial against *Helicobacter pylori* infections (such as peptic ulcers and gastritis), diabetic foot ulcers, post-surgical wounds... you name it, this honey can probably heal it.

Manuka honey is derived from the manuka bush – a shrub in the tea tree family, which is indigenous to New Zealand (with a close relative in some parts of Australia), and which only blooms for three weeks out of the year.

The science behind history's sweetest bacteria-buster

In order to fully grasp how manuka honey works, it helps to understand the antiseptic properties of ordinary honey first. These are due to several factors. The first of these is honey's osmotic – or water-withdrawing – effect. Not only does its ability to draw fluid from tissues give wounds a moist healing environment (absolutely necessary for new tissue growth) but it also draws harmful bacteria out and away from the point of infection.

Moreover, honey's fructose and glucose molecules interact strongly with water, leaving very few H_2O molecules 'free'. This inhibits the growth of the many strains of bacteria that require interaction with water in order to multiply. Nevertheless, there are still strains of bacteria that thrive under such conditions – so this quality alone can't offer complete protection.

Another healing aspect of ordinary honey is its acidity. The ideal pH range for the sustained growth of most pathogens is between 7.2 and 7.4. With a pH of between 3.2 and 4.5, however, the environment that honey creates around a wound is effectively hostile toward bacteria. But unfortunately, when diluted by bodily fluids of a higher pH, honey's natural acidity is reduced, preventing it from reaching deeper tissue and making for a much less reliable antibacterial agent.

The third and most noteworthy element of honey's curative ability is its hydrogen peroxide content that is produced after bees secrete glucose oxidase into the nectar. However, the antibacterial capabilities of this hydrogen peroxide are short-lived, as during the process of maturation the honey's acidity will cause the hydrogen peroxide to decompose by rendering glucose oxidase virtually inactive. For this reason, full-strength honey does not offer significant protection from bacteria.

Honey more effective than many cough medicines

New research from the US suggests that naturally-occurring honey may ease coughs and respiratory illnesses in children more effectively than many over-the-counter medicines.

During the trial, scientists from the Penn State College of Medicine asked parents to give either honey, honey-flavoured dextromethorphan (DM), or no treatment to 105 children, between the ages of two and 18 children, all suffering from nocturnal coughs.

The trial was partially blind, researchers said, as parents could not distinguish between the honey and the medication, although those administering no medication were aware of this fact.

The parents were asked to report on cough frequency and severity, how bothersome the cough was, and how well both adult and child slept, both 24 hours before and during the night of the dosage.

According to researcher Ian Paul, all the parents indicated that honey yielded the greatest improvement, followed by DM, while no treatment was consistently named as the poorest treatment. Based on parental 'symptom points', children treated with honey improved by an average of 10.71 points compared with 8.39 points for DM-treated children and 6.41 points for those who were not treated.

This is promising news as over-the-counter cough and cold medicines can have potentially harmful side effects in children, such as dystonic reactions, severe involuntary muscle contractions and spasms.

All things considered, there's no doubt that honey is a great thing to keep around the house for minor cuts or burns – and even for treating more serious conditions if handled correctly – but its limitations are also pretty clear. An ointment for stubborn post-surgical wounds and severe bedsores would have to be leaps and bounds more powerful – not to mention stable enough as to be impervious to outside factors such as temperature, light, moisture and age. And that's where the phytochemicals in manuka honey set it apart.

Manuka honey succeeds where other types of honey fail

Unlike other varieties of honey, manuka has an additional anti-bacterial property that isn't attributable to acidity, osmolarity, or the activity of hydrogen peroxide – evidenced primarily by its being twice as effective as other forms of honey against certain types of aggressive bacteria, including *E. coli* and MRSA (*J Appl Bacteriol. 1992 Nov; 73(5): 388-94*).

One of its advantages is that dilution doesn't affect its antibacterial activity, so all of its original acidity is spared. It also doesn't require oxygen – making it ideal for dressings and the cavities of deep wounds. And most importantly, its activity is unaffected by the enzymes present in wound fluid – which is one of the major shortcomings of other types of honey in this context (*J Pharm Pharmacol. 1991 Dec; 43(12): 817-22*).

Manuka honey also has other health benefits – including an ability to help combat gastric ulcers. A study performed by Professor of Biochemistry Dr Molan and his team at The Honey Research Unit at the University of Waikato in New Zealand, showed that five different biopsies of gastric ulcers all responded positively when exposed to a solution consisting of 20 per cent manuka honey. A 40 per cent solution of another type of honey (the antibacterial activity of which relied on hydrogen peroxide alone) elicited no response at all (*J R Soc Med. 1994 Jan; 87(1): 9-12*).

Further research has revealed that a solution consisting of as little as 5 per cent active manuka is still capable of delivering significant protection – most likely, the research team concluded, due to the inhibition of *Helicobacter pylori*, something which may explain one of honey's traditional uses as a treatment for dyspepsia.

In another study conducted over a 21-day trial period, 30 volunteers were assigned to chew or suck on either sugarless gum or a chewable form of manuka honey for 10 minutes, three times a day, in order to assess the possible effects the honey might have on gingivitis and plaque. At the end of the trial, both plaque scores and bleeding sites were significantly reduced in the manuka group. No significant changes were noted in the control group (*J Int Acad Periodontol. 2004 Apr; 6(2): 63-7*).

To benefit from manuka honey, take two to three teaspoonfuls (10-15g) before meals.

Roasted veg with manuka honey and feta cheese

This recipe serves 4-6 people

For this dish you will need the following ingredients:

2 red peppers, chopped
2 carrots, chopped
500g baby courgettes, chopped
2 red onions, each cut into 4 chunks
½ butternut squash, peeled and cut into chunks
6 tbsp extra virgin olive oil
4 sprigs thyme
200g feta cheese
3 to 4 tbsp manuka honey

To prepare:

Preheat the oven to 200C/400F/Gas Mark 6.
Place all the vegetables in a large roasting tin with the olive oil. Season, add the thyme, then roast for about 40 minutes.

Cut the feta cheese into cubes and add to the vegetables. Gently stir through with the honey. Return to the oven for another five minutes before serving.

CHAPTER 13

Sugar – How too much can increase your risk of a stroke, heart attack and diabetes

Unfortunately, in the West we have a tendency to overindulge on sweet sugary foods, which has been linked to the massive increase in obesity and Type 2 diabetes.

For this reason you should only eat sugary foods in moderation – that includes the sugar-containing recipes in this book (they're intended for special treats and not for regular consumption! Better still, try substituting them with honey, apple juice or dried fruit in desserts and cakes instead).

Studies have linked sugar to increasing the risk of circulatory diseases, such as atherosclerosis and stroke. It is thought that this has a lot to do with how the liver responds to sugar and insulin.

Each time you eat, insulin is released into your bloodstream, which pushes glucose into your muscle cells for energy production. In addition, insulin stops your liver from releasing fats into your bloodstream. This is necessary because, just after a meal, the enzymes that break down fats are busy dealing with the fat from the food you have just eaten.

Scientists have recently discovered how this process can go wrong (*J. Nutrition 131: 2074, 2001*). Frequent, low-fat, high-carb snacks – which are loaded with sugar – expose your liver to high levels of insulin for long periods without a break. This appears to flick a metabolic switch in your liver, which stimulates it to release large amounts of fat into your bloodstream. High blood fat levels cause the formation of 'very low density lipoprotein' (VLDL), also called 'bad cholesterol', which sticks to the sides of your arteries and narrows them – increasing your risk of heart disease or stroke.

High blood fat levels also start a vicious cycle that leads, ultimately to diabetes. First, they block insulin receptors on your muscle cells, making them 'insulin resistant'. This means that glucose can't enter your cells, causing your pancreas to produce more insulin in an effort to bring blood sugar levels down. Glucose is then diverted to your fat cells, which become overloaded – leading to weight gain. Eventually these become insulin resistant, too, leaving no route for glucose to be taken out of your bloodstream. The overloaded fat cells flood your bloodstream with fatty acids, which start killing the insulin-secreting cells in your pancreas. This results in full Type 2 diabetes, with daily insulin injections needed to keep you alive.

The simple sugar, fructose, also has a detrimental effect on your liver, and studies have shown that a high fructose diet causes a significant rise in blood fats (*Am. J. Clin. Nutr. 72(5): 1128-34, 2000*). Alarmingly, since the 1970s, food manufacturers have used corn syrup, which is almost pure fructose, as a cheap sweetener in processed foods – even in so-called 'healthy' low-fat meals – to make them more palatable. This new research emphasises the importance of following a diet that excludes sugar and is low in refined carbohydrates.

Flavonoids found in dark chocolate help lower high blood pressure

Eating dark chocolate may help lower blood pressure, boost normal responses to insulin to keep blood sugar levels down, and improve blood vessel function in patients with high blood pressure, according to new research findings. All of these effects would be expected to decrease the risk of heart attack and stroke.

The study, published by the American Heart Association (AHA), joins a growing body of research that show compounds found in chocolate called flavonoids can help the blood vessels work more smoothly, perhaps reducing the risk of heart disease.

Flavonoids are a class of water-soluble plant pigments. While they are not considered essential nutrients, some flavonoids help strengthen capillaries and other connective tissue, and some function as anti-inflammatory, antihistaminic and antiviral agents.

"Previous studies suggest flavonoid-rich foods, including fruits, vegetables, tea, red wine and chocolate, might offer cardiovascular benefits, but this is one of the first clinical trials to look specifically at dark chocolate's effect on lowering blood pressure among people with hypertension," said Jeffrey Blumberg of Tufts University, Boston, in the US, who led the study.

This study suggests that cocoa flavonoids appear to have benefits on vascular function and glucose sensitivity. Blumberg and colleagues at the University of L'Aquila in Italy studied 10 men and 10 women with high blood pressure. For 15 days, half ate a daily 3.5 ounce (100 gram) bar of specially formulated, flavonoid-rich dark chocolate, while the other half ate the same amount of white chocolate (*Hypertension 2005; 46: 398*).

Then each group 'crossed over' and ate the other chocolate. White chocolate was selected for comparison because, unlike dark chocolate, it does not contain flavonoids. However, it does contain all the other ingredients and calories found in dark chocolate.

Blumberg's team found that when the volunteers ate the dark chocolate, they had a 12mm Hg decrease in systolic blood pressure (the top number in a blood pressure reading) and a 9mm Hg decrease in diastolic blood pressure (the bottom number) on average. Blood pressure did not change when the volunteers ate white chocolate.

Eating dark chocolate also seemed to improve how the body used insulin, and reduced low density lipoprotein (LDL) or 'bad' cholesterol by about 10 per cent on average. So while the study used a specially formulated, flavonoid-rich dark chocolate, it is clear that regular dark chocolate is a better choice to eat because neither white or milk chocolate have similar amounts of flavonoids as regular dark chocolate does.

Scientists are far from being able to make specific recommendations for patients based on their research on chocolate so far. Blumberg cautioned that you can't just add it on top of your diet. "It's still a high-calorie food. You don't want to have excess calories or put on weight if you have hypertension," Blumberg said. "But as part of a healthful diet, it is something that you can enjoy and not feel you are violating the principles of a healthful diet."

The indulgent dessert below is a delicious way to enjoy dark chocolate as an occasional treat.

Indulgent chocolate and walnut mousse

This recipe serves 6 people

For this dish you will need the following ingredients:

250g dark chocolate with a high cocoa content (approx. 70%)
75g butter
1 tsp honey
8 egg whites
4 egg yolks
300ml double cream
1 tsp icing sugar
75g walnuts

To prepare:

Break the chocolate into small pieces and place in a small bowl along with the butter. Place the bowl over the top of a saucepan of gently simmering water and stir until the chocolate melts.

Take about a third of the mixture and stir in a spoonful of honey and a splash of double cream to make a thick chocolate sauce.

Meanwhile, whisk the egg yolks into the remainder of the melted chocolate and set aside somewhere warm. In another mixing bowl, whisk the remainder of the cream until it is starting to thicken, be careful not to over whip the cream at this stage.

Fold about two thirds of the cream into the melted chocolate and place the remainder of the cream in the fridge.

Meanwhile, in yet another mixing bowl, whisk the egg whites and the icing sugar together until they are quite stiff.

Immediately fold half the egg white into the chocolate, only using a wooden spoon or a spatula to do this, as a whisk will let all the air escape resulting in quite a heavy dessert.

Fold the rest of the whites in until you have a really smooth chocolate mousse.

Using the chocolate sauce you made earlier, line the bottom of each glass with about 1cm. Fill each glass to the top with the chocolate mousse and place in the fridge to set.

On a flat baking tray evenly lay out the walnuts and place under a hot grill until they are nicely toasted on each side, you can do these in an oven also if you want. Do not take your eye off them as nuts burn quickly. Once toasted, crush them with a rolling pin or chop coarsely with a sharp knife.

Once the nuts have cooled slightly, fold them into the remainder of the whipped cream you kept from earlier.

Place a large dollop of the walnut cream on top of each dessert and drizzle with the rest of the chocolate sauce. Sprinkle any nuts that you have left over the top and serve.

CHAPTER 14

Why not all super foods are healthy for everyone

It is important to point out that the super foods outlined in *Super Foods for a Super Healthy You* should not be eaten by those with a food intolerance or allergy to them.

A 'food allergy' directly affects your immune system after eating a particular food. Your body produces antibodies, just as it would respond to a bacteria or virus. Every time the food is eaten a reaction occurs, which can be life threatening – as in cases of anaphylactic shock, whereby your tissues swell up, causing breathing difficulties and even heart failure. True allergies usually appear in childhood and rarely go away.

A food intolerance involves a 'bad reaction' to one or more foods. Symptoms include dark circles and puffiness under the eyes, fatigue, headaches, depression, digestive problems, diarrhoea, frequent infections, water retention, an inability to lose weight, swollen glands and chronic inflammation. They often develop later on in life, and factors such as stress and poor nutrition may be involved.

Up to 90% of migraines involve food sensitivities!

More than 30 medical conditions, such as peptic ulcers, kidney disease, epilepsy, asthma and chronic bronchitis, have been shown, in many cases, to involve food allergies. Many people with rheumatoid arthritis find their symptoms are diet-related, and research suggests that one in three sufferers could control this disease by eliminating allergies (*Lancet 338: 1209, 1991*). Milk, beef, wheat, corn, tomatoes, aubergines and sweet peppers are common culprits.

Most sufferers of irritable bowel syndrome (IBS) are sensitive to certain foods *(Lancet ii: 295-7, 1983)* and Crohn's disease (an inflammatory bowel disease) can also be aggravated by food sensitivities *(Lancet ii: 177-80, 1985)*. Both conditions usually involve a reaction to wheat, gluten, dairy products or yeast. And studies show that up to 90 per cent of migraines are caused by food sensitivities! *(Lancet ii: 865-9, 1983)*.

Conventional tests for detecting food allergies are often inaccurate

If you suspect you have a food allergy, your doctor can refer you for a skin test. Your skin is pricked, in contact with various substances, to see whether an inflammatory reaction occurs. Skin tests can be good for detecting allergies to airborne chemicals, but are not very accurate for diagnosing food allergies. Blood tests, which look for specific antibodies, are more reliable, but both tests will only pick up 'true food allergies' involving your immune system.

For food intolerances, the 'cytotoxic' test is often used – a blood sample is examined for any changes to your white blood cells, but its accuracy is 80 per cent at best. Non-invasive tests detect changes to your body's electrical energy field; electro-acupuncture measures these changes using a galvanometer, whilst kinesiology detects them through muscle resistance. The accuracy of both methods largely depends on the practitioners' skill.

Identify problems effectively with an elimination diet

The most reliable way of detecting food allergies is through an elimination diet. This involves avoiding all foods likely to cause allergies for at least two weeks, then reintroducing them one at a time. You should do this under the supervision of a nutritionist, who will assess your nutritional status before you start and monitor your progress.

Once you have identified the offending foods, keep them out of your diet. Typical foods include wheat, eggs, soya or milk. Unless you have a 'true allergy' to a food, you may be able to reintroduce it in small amounts after six months and continue to eat it occasionally.

The integrity of your gut mucosa – the layer of cells lining your gut – often underlies food allergies. It should be selective about what it lets into your bloodstream, to be transported to your liver. But if it becomes damaged, due to a yeast infection, medication, or poor diet, it can let undigested proteins through. This is called 'leaky gut syndrome', and can cause chronic diarrhoea, bloating and abdominal pain. The presence of these 'foreign' food molecules in your blood often triggers food allergy responses.

If you suspect you have a food allergy, see a nutritional therapist and follow an elimination diet. Maintain the health of your gut by avoiding sugar and refined carbohydrates, cutting down on coffee and alcohol, and eating plenty of fresh vegetables and essential fatty acids (from oily fish, nuts and seeds).

CHAPTER 15

Is organic food really better?

The answer to this really does seem to be a resounding yes. There are many health advantages to buying organic foods, plus it has never been easier now that there is an increased availability of fresh organic produce. More and more agricultural land is being turned over to organic production and more and more supermarket chains now stock a large range of organic produce.

Organic farming methods mean that crops are not subjected to pesticides, insecticides, fungicides and herbicides, which reduces the risk of toxicity. In addition, organic meat is a good way of ensuring that you are not consuming animals that have been given antibiotics to promote growth.

As well as having negative effects on health, these antibiotics increase the resistant strains of bacteria that are now rapidly appearing. It also means no hormones or other medicinal drugs will be present in the meat. Plus, from an animal welfare point of view, organic farming methods mean that animals are treated in a more natural and humane way.

Organic produce also means that fertilizers aren't being used, which deplete the soil of vital nutrients like selenium, zinc, magnesium and chromium. Currently in the UK organic foods also have to be free from genetically modified produce. Although the full potential risks from genetically modified foods has yet to be unveiled by research, there is a possibility that they may contain substances toxic to humans.

All genuinely organic food in the UK will be labelled as such and should carry the Soil Association symbol to show that it has been certified as organic. You may also see the term 'conservation grade' labelled on food products. This means the same as the organic label but shows that the farming practices used also employ additional measures to conserve the surrounding environment.

If you see the term 'transitional' labelled on a food item then this means that the food has come from a place where organic practices are being used but that it has not yet completed the full two-year change over period. To be certified as organic there are strict regulations and guidelines that must be followed, and there is a two-year conversion period when these principles are applied but the product cannot be labelled as organic until this time deadline has been reached.

While most of us choose organic foods usually because of what ISN'T in them – pesticides, growth hormones and antibiotics, just to name a few choice chemicals – new research suggests that we might get even more benefit from organically-grown fruits and vegetables because of what IS in them... a substance that might help protect us from heart attacks, strokes, and even cancer.

In a recent issue of the *British Journal of Nutrition*, researchers reported on their assessment of 35 different brands of vegetable soup, both organic and non-organic. They found that on average, the organic brands contained nearly six times as much salicylic acid, a natural anti-inflammatory agent.

The 11 organic brands tested boasted an average of 117 nanograms per gram of salicylic acid, while the 24 non-organic brands only contained an average of 20 ng/g. One soup in particular contained nearly 50 times the concentration of salicylic acid as in the average non-organic soup; the carrot and coriander soup from Scotland's Simply Organic contained 1040 ng/g.

Previous research has shown that salicylic acid can help fight atherosclerosis and certain types of cancer. More and more studies are suggesting that the body's inflammatory response plays a critical role in many types of chronic disease. And earlier work by the same British research team proved that eating salicylic-rich foods translates into higher blood concentrations of the acid, so there is substantial reason to add this new finding to organic produce's list of benefits.

The researchers theorise that organic fruits and vegetables contain more salicylic acid because plants produce the substance as a natural defence mechanism. Without pesticides and other chemicals to keep insects and disease at bay, organically grown plants must protect themselves in order to thrive. This may explain why these plants contain so much more of this beneficial acid.

This study shows that what Mother Nature puts INTO our foods is just as important as what she doesn't. And if you've been unsure whether there was enough benefit to pay the additional cost of organic, here's another reason to consider it. Many supermarket chains across the country now offer organic produce right next to the conventionally grown fruits and vegetables. In most cases, you don't have to go out of your way to eat organic anymore – but even if you do, this research shows us that the benefits are even greater than we thought.

CHAPTER 16

The way you cook your food can be just as important as the foods you opt for

W hile including more of certain foods in your diet can make a real difference to your health, energy levels and overall well-being, the way you cook and prepare foods is also important.

To make sure you're getting all the vital nutrients from your foods, it is important to know which cooking methods help to retain them and those that deplete them... and worse, can actually harm your health. The following guidelines are based on modern scientific research findings.

Make sure your cooking utensils and tap water aren't damaging your brain

Although nobody knows the exact cause of Alzheimer's disease, scientists have found that many Alzheimer's patients have excessive amounts of aluminium in their brains. It is now becoming more widely accepted that aluminium may play a major role in the development of the disease (*Can J Public Health 1992; 83: 97-100*).

Aluminium cookware was thought to be the source of this aluminium build-up. However, the puzzle for scientists was how the aluminium got into the brain, as aluminium is unable to cross your blood/brain barrier. The answer, it seems, may lie in tap water, particularly fluoridated tap water (for more information on fluoride's negative effects see page 215).

It is now thought that aluminium contained in cookware may become unstable in the presence of fluoridated water and released. Research has shown that boiling fluoridated tap water in an aluminium pan means the water absorbs almost 200 parts per million (ppm) of aluminium and up to 600 ppm with prolonged boiling.

This did not happen when non-fluoridated water was boiled in aluminium pans. The significance of this is that aluminium fluoride, a compound made from fluoride in water and the aluminium in pans, does pass the blood/brain barrier, which was previously believed to be impossible.

Laboratory tests conducted by Dr Julie Varner and her team at the Bryan Alzheimer's Disease Research Center at Duke University in North Carolina have confirmed this – that the action of aluminium and fluoride in water can result in pre-senile dementia and kidney damage (*Neuroscience Research Communications, 1993, 13:2, 99-104, Society for Neuroscience Annual Meeting; San Diego, CA, 1995, Brain Research 1998; 784: 284-298*). Age-related conditions resulted with both aluminium/fluoride-laced water and water containing both sodium fluoride and aluminium fluoride.

You may think you're not at risk if your pots and pans aren't made of aluminium. But how many of your pots and pans are non-stick? When non-stick surfaces were used on aluminium pans, it was believed that this would insulate the metal and stop it from coming into direct contact with food. But the non-stick materials, Teflon and Tefal, are made from the polymer poly-tetra-fluoro-ethylene (PTFE). And the 'F' stands for 'fluorine'.

PTFE is harmless when cold. However, the 19 July 2001 issue of *Nature* highlighted the dangers posed by Teflon when heated, after fluorine was detected (*Nature 2001; 412: 312-324*). So, despite the fact that Teflon is perceived by many as being safer, it could in fact be a significant source of fluoride pollution at normal cooking temperatures – and have a detrimental effect on the brain.

The bottom line is that there are strong grounds to suspect that, where a source of fluorine can combine with aluminium this may increase the risk of Alzheimer's disease. It may not be merely coincidence that the world's most fluoridated country, Ireland, has a massive 30,000 cases of Alzheimer's out of a total population of three million. And while Teflon was believed to reduce the danger, its fluoride content may actually increase it.

Under the circumstances, at least until more is proved about this terrible disease and its causes, you may wish to consider throwing out that aluminium cookware – non-stick or not – in favour of stainless steel or cast-iron cookware.

Microwaves: They're convenient, they're fast, but are they really safe?

This is a frequently-asked question, especially as in the last 10 years or so, microwave cooking has become immensely popular. But do you really know what the microwave process does to your food, and how it affects the food value? Does the excessive heat destroy the vitamin content?

These are important questions to which there are no concrete answers to as yet. There are very few studies on microwave cooking and food quality. What studies do exist are all bad news for microwaving – they universally describe some type of damage. One study conducted in Switzerland in 1991 by Hertel and Blanc, of the Swiss Federal Institute of Technology and the University Institute for Biochemistry, showed breakdown of vitamin B12 to inactive degradation products in microwaved foods.

Russian research concerning neurological effects of altered magnetic states of microwaved foods caused the Russian government to outlaw all food microwave apparatus in 1976 (this law was lifted after Perestroika). Another study reported in the US journal *Pediatrics* (vol. 89, no. 4, April 1992) showed depletion of antibodies and breakdown of enzymes when breast milk is microwaved.

There's also a problem with release of potentially toxic molecules into the food from packaging designed to help brown food during microwaving. This includes items such as pizza, chips, waffles, popcorn and breaded fish – and these findings were determined by the Food and Drug Association.

The most controlled (and scary) research was almost stopped from anyone knowing about it before being published. Hertel and Blanc (mentioned above) conducted another study where participants were observed under close scrutiny and blood tested after randomly eating food that was either microwaved or conventionally cooked.

They found all sorts of potentially nasty stuff: (1) Blood haemoglobin levels decreased significantly after ingesting microwaved foods, both total levels and the amount contained in each red blood cell; (2) White blood cell levels tended to increase for no other reason than foods were microwaved; (3) Microwaves altered protein molecules; (4) LDL cholesterol (the 'bad' type) increased relative to HDL cholesterol (the 'good' type).

The problem was, they were immediately sued by the 'Swiss Association of Dealers for Electroapparatuses for Households and Industry', and one of the authors was convicted by the Swiss Federal Court of 'interfering with commerce'. The fine was the equivalent of around £40,000. So, the message is you think twice before stepping on too many big-money toes. However you look at it, there appears to be a problem with those high frequency, alternating current (meaning abnormal for the human system) electromagnetic waves.

Another disadvantage of using microwaves is their tendency to heat foods unevenly, indicating that some of the food is not sufficiently heated to kill all the bacteria or parasites that might be present. This uneven heating also creates hot spots in food that may release synthetic oestrogens found in certain plastics.

But even when using only glass (Pyrex) containers, low levels of radiation escaping from microwave ovens may still be harmful, and you should exercise caution when standing in front of a microwave unit while it's in use. Until we have more definitive studies available, it would seem that the safest use of microwaves may be as a cooking aid (for defrosting, heating liquids, etc.) rather than as a method for primary cooking.

CHAPTER 17

Drink your way to good health

According to research findings, what you drink can have just as important health implications as what you eat. The health advantages and disadvantages of various beverages are outlined in the next section to help you make the right choices when it comes to quenching your thirst.

Water can affect the amount of nutrients your body's getting from the food you eat

The importance of drinking adequate amounts of water can't be stressed enough. Water helps to flush harmful toxins from your system.

In fact, water is more important to the body than any other nutrient and can help prevent many chronic diseases, yet most people don't realise that they are actually deficient in it. It's so commonplace that most people take it for granted and don't drink nearly as much of it as they should to maintain good health. Unless your body is properly hydrated, you won't experience the full benefits to be had from eating a healthy diet.

Think of your garden after a long summer drought... the earth is baked hard and your plants are wilting. Would you sprinkle fertiliser straight onto the dry ground, or would you water the garden well first, so that the fertiliser could do its job properly? Like a parched garden, your body won't be able to blossom without enough water.

You may be thinking, "But I can't be dehydrated; I drink a lot and I rarely feel thirsty." But if you drink tea, coffee, cola or alcoholic drinks, their diuretic effect (increasing the frequency of urination) is actually robbing your body of more water than they provide. One of the most insidious effects of this low level dehydration is that it causes the thirst signal in your brain to 'switch off', so you don't feel thirsty.

Other factors that cause dehydration include chocolate and sugary foods, salty snacks, highly processed foods, artificial additives and tobacco smoke. Air conditioning, air travel, computer screens and watching television all contribute to dehydration too.

What happens when you are dehydrated? Your body is designed to survive temporary water shortages by conserving and rationing available water. When you're dehydrated, however, your body reduces urine and sweat production and extracts more water from the contents of your colon – a common cause of constipation.

Your body also becomes less able to eliminate poisonous waste products, resulting in headaches, lethargy and bad breath. If the kidneys, skin and colon are not eliminating these wastes properly, more strain is put onto your liver to detoxify them. Most people actually need to rid their bodies of waste products more than they need to get extra nutrients in.

The longer your body remains dehydrated, the greater the risk of serious problems developing. A dehydrated body produces increased amounts of both histamine and cholesterol. Increased amounts of histamine promote inflammation, pain and allergies. Cholesterol gets deposited in your arteries – increasing your risk of heart disease or stroke. Other serious health problems – which may be due in part to severe dehydration – include chronic fatigue syndrome, peptic ulcers, high blood pressure, hardening of the arteries, arthritis, back pain, asthma and diabetes.

Drinking two litres of water a day is the biggest step you can take to reverse dehydration. To fully rehydrate your body eat plenty of foods with a high water content such as salad, vegetables, cooked pulses and tofu. However, you should avoid drinking anything other than small sips of water when you are eating in order to facilitate good digestion.

Rehydrating your body will make you look and feel healthier. You may even find that symptoms that have plagued you for years mysteriously disappear.

How to make sure you're getting 8 glasses (2 litres) of water a day

- Drink two glasses of water when you wake up in the morning – after all you've just gone 8 hours without fluids.
- Drink two glasses of water before going to bed (although those with weak bladders may want to cut back on this in the interest of getting a good night's rest).
- Drink a glass of water half an hour before you eat and then drink another two hours after the meal.
- Drink whenever you feel thirsty.

Make sure water isn't making you ill

Two recent studies from Idaho in the US and Canada bring important warnings for the millions of people who enjoy their water in convenient plastic bottles. First the good news: bottled water is not bad for you. But you may be surprised to find out that what you do with the bottle after you've drained it might lead to serious health problems, if you then use the same bottle to refill it with more water.

Researchers from the University of Calgary collected water samples from 76 plastic bottles used by students in a Calgary elementary school. About one third of the samples contained bacterial contamination severe enough that, had the water come from a tap, health officials would have issued a 'boil water' advisory. Some samples even contained faecal coliforms (bacteria which are excreted in faeces). Their presence in water is used as a broad indicator of the extent of water contamination by faecal material.

Cathy Ryan, the lead professor of the study, noted that if faecal coliforms were found in a town water supply, it would have to be shut down.

These contamination problems are a direct result of reusing water bottles without proper washing between each use. The researchers speculated that the contamination of the elementary school water bottles was likely complicated by insufficient hygiene – specifically, a lack of thorough hand washing. Nevertheless, any water bottle reused again and again without washing is subject to contamination with bacteria.

Cleanliness doesn't guarantee safety

A University of Idaho survey revealed that the reuse of water and soft water drink bottles was widespread on the UI campus, with some individuals using a single bottle for several weeks. One participant reported that he had reused the same bottle for six months. This survey was taken in conjunction with a graduate programme study that examined the effects of repeated bottle use.

The UI study tested water samples from typical soft-drink and water bottles made from a plastic called polyethylene terephthalate (PET).

Analysis of the samples showed that with repeated use, toxic chemicals in the plastic can break down and migrate into the liquid inside. One of the toxins that appeared with regularity was di(2-ethylhexyl) adipate, a carcinogen that has been shown to cause liver damage and reproductive problems.

Furthermore, when bottles were used repeatedly, the concentration of toxins gradually became more pronounced. And ironically, washing the bottles didn't help – in fact it only made matters worse. The UI data suggested that the breakdown of toxins was accelerated by regular exposure to hot water and soap.

Rotate!

So the water bottle dilemma has some similarity to the problem with tap water. Lead in water pipes is drawn into the water just as the toxins in plastic are drawn into the bottled water. The difference, of course, is that you have far more control with bottled water. And in most cases, bottled water is less contaminated than tap water.

As these studies demonstrate, it's probably not a good idea to stick with one bottle for very long – even if you clean it after each use. A fresh bottle every couple of days would seem to be the wise way to quench your thirst.

Of course, you can always take your water the old-fashioned way... in a glass.

Fluoride

While the merits of water cannot be rated too highly, it is important that you use a water filter or drink bottled water. The reason for this is to help minimise the fluoride content of the water you may be drinking. Fluoridation has been a contentious subject for decades... only now is the full story about this invisible enemy finally emerging.

Fluoride is an odourless, colourless substance but despite these innocent-sounding attributes it is anything but. The fluoride used in water fluoridation projects is actually a toxic by-product of the fertiliser industry. There are now a growing number of studies linking fluoride consumption to serious conditions such as osteoporosis, genetic and cognitive disorders, and even cancer (*Fluoride 1995; 28(4): 189-92; Fluoride 1996; 29: 190-2*).

Its supporters, including the British Dental Association, claim that fluoride helps strengthen teeth and prevents dental cavities. Yet far from protecting teeth there is now mounting evidence to suggest that it can harm them instead, leading to dental fluorosis in children. Fluorosis causes unsightly white, yellow or brown spots on teeth and can eventually destroy them (*J Am Dent Assoc 1936; 23: 574*).

It's not just water that can be source of fluoride it is also present in many toothpastes, mouthwashes, canned foods and even tea bags.

Follow these 7 steps to protect your health against fluoride's harmful effects

1. If you live in a fluoridated area get a reverse osmosis filter fitted to the main kitchen tap. For more information contact The Pure H2O Company on 01784 221180, or visit: www.purewater.co.uk

2. Alternatively you can help minimise the risk by drinking filtered or bottled water.

3. Use a non-fluoride toothpaste and mouthwash. Fluoride-free toothpaste brands include Boot's Non-Fluoride, Tom's, Tea Tree, and Weleda.

4. Try to be aware of the fluoride content of food and drink – tinned fruit, vegetables and drinks are especially high. Fluoride is present in tea, regardless of whether it's made with fluoridated water or not. So, opt for herbal teas made from non-fluoridated water instead.

5. Eat foods low in fluoride, such as eggs, milk, red meats (not organs), and fruit with protective rinds (such as lemons, bananas and pineapples).

---

6. Supplementing with calcium and magnesium salts helps eliminate fluoride from your body.
7. Avoid using kitchen utensils with non-stick coatings such as Teflon – these are made of fluoride.

Coffee: Is your morning cup making you feel rundown and ill-tempered?

Coffee is a powerful stimulant that is extremely addictive and has a dehydrating effect. In addition it can stress your adrenal glands, causing them to become underactive over time, which can leave you feeling 'burnt out'.

This can result in a range of debilitating symptoms like an inability to concentrate, headaches, excessive fatigue and weakness, nervousness, irritability, depression and insomnia. In terms of insomnia you should bear in mind that the effects of caffeine last for up to 20 hours – so even having a strong cup of coffee in the morning could keep you awake at night.

It also causes fluctuations in blood sugar levels. A Dutch study that examined the effects of caffeine on insulin sensitivity revealed that moderate caffeine intake may decrease insulin sensitivity by as much as 15 per cent – so increasing the risk of Type 2 diabetes (*Diabetes Care, 25: 364-369, 2002*).

However, it's not all bad news on the coffee front...

Coffee berries and pomegranates – The unusual duo that together provide superior antioxidant action

There's good news for those of you who enjoy a cup or two of freshly brewed coffee in the mornings. Putting aside its high caffeine content and dehydrating effect for one moment, coffee is able to provide benefits that extend beyond simply waking you up and increasing your mental acuity. It has been found to lower the risk of Parkinson's disease, gallstones, Type 2 diabetes and colon cancer.

However, some of coffee's greatest health benefits are being discarded before it ever makes its way into your favourite mug. These benefits aren't coming from those deliciously aromatic roasted beans. Before they were cooked, bagged, and ground for local cafes and supermarkets – before they were even harvested from the plant, in fact – the beans were cloaked by one of the most powerful (and least-known) antioxidants on the planet: the coffee fruit.

Due to its high perishability, this bright red outer layer (also called the cherry by coffee growers) is normally thrown away in favour of its insides. At present Van Drunen Farms, a family-owned business in the US, is the only supplier of whole coffee fruit around. They've dubbed it the coffee berry – and today, thanks to new patent-pending technology, product developers can get it in the form of a whole powder or a concentrated extract, skirting the problem of spoilage altogether.

This has led to the development of a ground-breaking new supplement called CoffeeGranate Forte that packs double the antioxidant punch by combining the benefits of coffee berries with the incredible power of pomegranates – the numerous benefits of which we featured earlier on page 39.

Packed full of health-giving ingredients that help deliver oxygen to your cells

One of the main reasons coffee berries are so beneficial is due to their geographical origins – these include Columbia, Costa Rica, Brazil, and other parts of Central and South America. Coffee bushes thrive in the fertile volcanic soil these mountainous areas provide – it's loaded with nutrients and minerals, all of which are absorbed by the plant as it grows.

The abundance of phytochemicals produced by the coffee berries that grow on these bushes is also reliant upon the bright, hot, uninhibited rays of the sun. Being so close to the equator these countries have much higher levels of UV radiation. This low latitude, in combination with the high altitudes at which the coffee plant grows, means that the by-products of photosynthesis not only furnish its unique nutritional needs, but also serve as a protective mechanism against its unrelenting exposure to the sun.

The final result is a fruit enriched with a powerful blend of health-promoting, free radical-fighting polyphenols that you'll only find in plants native to consistently sun-soaked climates.

Among these polyphenols are proanthocyanidins, a group of flavonoids found in a variety of plants and fruits – especially grape skins, which is why high amounts are found in red wine. White wine is not such a good source because the skins of the grapes are removed early during the production process. As you may already know by now, a large body of research has demonstrated these flavonoids' ability to support heart health, strengthen blood vessels, maintain joint flexibility, and uphold optimal metabolic processes in your body, including the delivery of oxygen to your cells.

Another big source of health benefits is the mix of mono-, oligo-, and polysaccharides you'll find intact in the coffee berry – many of which are otherwise destroyed in the roasting process of your typical coffee beans. Recent research has shown that, besides being a necessary source of fuel for your body, a certain family of these nutritive carbohydrates plays an especially crucial role in healthy biological signalling within your body – thereby reinforcing a strong and efficient immune system.

But perhaps the most important of the plant metabolites found in coffee berries are phenolic acids, also present in many other brightly coloured berries, like blueberries, strawberries and raspberries – all of which are well known in the nutritional world for their superior antioxidant power. As is the case in these berries, the particular compounds in coffee berry (including caffeic, chlorogenic, and ferulic acid) also happen to be adept at keeping free radicals at bay, while promoting proper cell division and – as an added perk – keeping sun-exposed skin looking young and healthy.

Get once-a-day defence made from equal parts pomegranate

As already mentioned, pomegranates are one of the hottest natural ingredients in the nutrition industry today, with a growing body of studies supporting their ability to, among other things, scavenge for free radicals (thereby promoting healthy cell division), keep your cardiovascular system strong, protect a healthy prostate, ease the transition of menopause, and – according to some of the most recent research – even preserve mental acuity.

Each daily serving of CoffeeGranate Forte includes 150mg of whole pomegranate extract standardized to 40 per cent punicosides, including punicalin and punicalagins (the ellagitannins that are the active ingredients responsible for over half of the fruit's antioxidant capacity).

One capsule is the equivalent of the 40ml to 50ml of pure pomegranate juice that has yielded significant health benefits in so many studies – but without all of the sugar and calories.

In addition to pomegranates, each serving of CoffeeGranate Forte provides 150mg of coffee fruit extract, standardized to 50 per cent phenolic acids – once again, among the most active phytochemicals in the coffee berry – to deliver the strongest antioxidant power possible.

It goes without saying that these two ingredients taken together make for an unbeatable combination. But just to put it into perspective for you, CoffeeGranate Forte registers in at a whopping 6,574 units per gram on the oxygen radical absorbence capacity (better known as ORAC) scale. On a gram-for-gram basis, that figure is hundreds of times higher than the same amount of fresh strawberries, raspberries, or even blueberries – and all at a serving size of just one capsule a day.

Research has discovered how coffee can help reduce the risk of alcohol-related pancreatitis

Pancreatitis is a condition in which the pancreas becomes inflamed, causing severe abdominal pain. The pancreas is a gland that lies behind your stomach and guts. It produces enzymes and hormones that help break down food and also help control blood sugar levels.

There are two types of pancreatitis: acute and chronic. In acute attacks, the inflammation comes on quickly and will usually go away leaving no permanent damage. In the UK, approximately two people in every 100,000 experience acute pancreatitis every year according to the NHS.

Chronic pancreatitis often starts as bouts of acute pancreatitis but eventually becomes a permanent condition. The NHS also found that each year, about one in every 100,000 people in the UK develops chronic pancreatitis.

Both kinds are often triggered by alcohol consumption which causes digestive enzymes to digest part of the pancreas. But now, scientists at the University of Liverpool have found out how coffee can reduce the risk of alcohol-induced pancreatitis (*"Scientists discover how coffee can reduce risk of pancreatitis"* University of Liverpool press *release, 13/03/06*).

Scientists have known for some time that coffee can reduce the risk of alcoholic pancreatitis, but have been unable to determine how. Professor Ole Petersen and Professor Robert Sutton, from the University's Physiological Laboratory and Division of Surgery, have found that cells in the pancreas can be damaged by alcohol and fat formed in the pancreas when oxygen levels in the organ are low.

Under these conditions, excessive amounts of calcium are released from stores within the cells of the pancreas. The mitochondria, which normally allows calcium to be pumped out of the cells, also becomes damaged. The excess calcium ends up destroying the pancreas cells.

Professor Petersen explains: "The primary cause of the build-up in calcium concentration is the movement of calcium stored inside the cells into the cell water through special channels. We have found that caffeine, present in drinks such as coffee, can at least partially close these channels. This explains why coffee consumption can reduce the risk of alcoholic pancreatitis. The caffeine effect, however, is weak and excessive coffee intake has its own dangers..."

While coffee is not the cure for pancreatitis, it can offer a way for you to help reduce the risk. If you do suffer from alcohol-related pancreatitis, unfortunately, the best thing that you can do for your health is to give up drinking.

Tea: Numerous benefits linked to your morning cup of tea

Here are just a few good reasons to put the kettle on...

... Drinking tea can boost your immunity and help protect you from disease

A report published in the early online edition of *The Proceedings of the National Academy of Sciences* (http://www.pnas.org/) has revealed that drinking tea can trigger a strong immune response in humans.

Both black and green teas contain an amino acid called L-theanine, which is a precursor to non-peptide alkylamine antigens that are also found in bacteria, parasites, fungi and tumour cells. Exposure to this antigen results in a memory response by the immune system, which then prepares itself to launch an attack on one of these pathogens (disease-causing microbes).

In a recent study, 11 volunteers were asked to drink five to six cups of black tea (containing a total of 2.2 micromoles of L-theanine) daily for two or four weeks. A control group was instructed to drink the same amount of instant coffee. Blood samples were taken at the start of the study and at the end of each week. In the group that received tea, gamma-delta T cells (involved in immune response) showed a greater ability to produce natural chemicals that combat disease after just two weeks. This benefit was not observed in the gamma-delta T cells of the coffee drinkers.

The authors conclude that: "Dietary intake of tea... may provide natural resistance to microbial infections and perhaps tumours."

... Drinking tea could lower your risk of bile stones and cancer

According to a population-based study in China, drinking at least one cup of tea a day could significantly reduce the risk of cancer in the gallbladder and bile ducts and reduce the risk of bile stones (*International Journal of Cancer, June 2006, Vol. 118, pp. 3089-3094*).

This finding adds to the growing list of benefits linked to tea and tea extracts – particularly the catechin extract, epigallocatechin gallate (EGCG) – to reducing the risk of Alzheimer's, certain cancers, as well as playing a role in weight loss.

The researchers, led by Ann Hsing from the US National Cancer Institute, assessed the demographic, medical and dietary histories of 627 people with bile tract cancers, 1,037 people with bile stones, and 959 randomly selected healthy controls.

The sample population was based in Shanghai, China, where the incidence of these types of cancers is reported to have increased in recent years. Although cancers of the gallbladder and bile ducts are relatively rare in the UK, they are highly fatal so it is important to find effective ways of preventing them.

Tea drinkers were defined by the researchers as anyone who drank at least one cup of tea per day for at least half a year.

"Among women, tea drinking was associated with lower risks of gallbladder and bile duct cancers and of biliary stones," reported the researchers. Specifically, women tea drinkers reduced their risk of gallbladder cancer by 44 per cent, bile duct cancer by 35 per cent and bile stones by 27 per cent.

For men, no significant association was observed between tea drinking and a lowered risk of developing these conditions. Hsing and her colleagues believe that these results may have been affected by the high number of smokers amongst the men, which may affect the incidence of these types of cancers.

"These findings add to the accumulating epidemiological evidence linking tea consumption with a lower risk of various cancers, particularly of the digestive tract," said the researchers.

The mechanism by which tea exerts a benefit is not clear, said the scientists, but "may involve anti-proliferative and anti-inflammatory properties of tea polyphenols, in particular EGCG." The researchers also mention that a plausible explanation may be due to effects of EGCG on oestrogen biosynthesis and other hormonal processes, which may help explain the benefits observed in women and not men.

The researchers called for future studies to replicate these results in other populations, as well as focusing research on determining the hormonal or other mechanisms involved.

... Green and black tea could play an important role in the prevention of Alzheimer's disease

Researchers from the University of Newcastle-upon-Tyne have discovered that drinking green and black tea can improve memory and could have potential as future treatments for Alzheimer's disease (*Phytotherapy Research, August 2004*).

The two are very similar – green tea consists of leaves from the plant Camilla sinensis, which, when fermented, is known as black tea. Dr Ed Okello of Newcastle University's Medicinal Plant Research Centre and colleagues conducted experiments using coffee, black tea and green tea.

They found that black and green tea both inhibited an enzyme called acetylcholinesterase, which breaks down a neurotransmitter called acetylcholine – an important compound that facilitates the transmission of messages between nerve cells, and which has been found to be deficient in sufferers of Alzheimer's disease. The researchers found that coffee had no effect on acetylcholinesterase.

The scientists also discovered that tea inhibited another enzyme known as butyrylcholinesterase, which is found in protein deposits in the brains of people with Alzheimer's disease. Additionally, green tea inhibited the enzyme beta-secretase for one week, whereas black tea was effective for only one day. Beta-secretase is an enzyme that initiates the formation of the protein amyloid in early Alzheimer's disease.

Dr Okello suggested that drinking tea could help improve memory and stated: "Although there is no cure for Alzheimer's, tea could potentially be another weapon in the armoury which is used to treat this disease and slow down its development.

"It would be wonderful if our work could help improve the quality of life for millions of sufferers and their carers. Our findings are particularly exciting as tea is already a very popular drink, it is inexpensive, and there do not seem to be any adverse side effects when it is consumed."

... More evidence regarding green tea's ability to lower the incidence of memory impairment

Most people believe that part of the natural process of ageing is a mild loss in memory or cognitive function. It might be as simple as forgetting what you went to the store to get, or what day and time your favourite TV programme is on.

Mild cognitive impairment (MCI) is a relatively recent term, used to describe people who have some problems with their memory but do not actually have dementia.

The Alzheimer's Society estimates that about 15 per cent of people in the UK experience MCI. However, MCI can lead to a higher risk of developing dementia or Alzheimer's, so it is important if you are experiencing problems with your memory that you see your doctor and get an accurate diagnosis.

There are different reasons why people may have some mild problems with their memory. As we mentioned above, some people will be in the early stages of Alzheimer's disease or another dementia. Others, however, will have MCI as a result of stress, anxiety, depression, physical illness or just an 'off day'.

So making sure we take steps to minimize stress, anxiety and are in good health are good ways to help avoid MCI. But a new study shows us that there is another thing we can do: drink green tea.

Researchers from the Tohoku University Graduate School of Medicine in Sendai, Japan found that people who drank more green tea had a lower occurrence of cognitive impairment (*Am J Clin Nutr 2006; 83(2): 355-61*).

Lead researcher, Shinichi Kuriyama and colleagues evaluated data from 1,002 volunteers aged 70 and over who participated in the Japanese Comprehensive Geriatric Assessment in 2002.

The men and women filled out questionnaires indicating how much they drank green tea, black tea and coffee. They then also underwent cognitive function tests that indicated whether they had no impairment, slight impairment, impairment or severe impairment.

The researchers discovered that those who drank two or more cups of green tea a day had a lower prevalence of cognitive impairment than people who drank three cups a week or less. If you don't like drinking that much tea, even people in the study who drank just one cup a day (or four to six a week) experienced about a 38 per cent reduction. The scientists didn't find a significant association between black tea or coffee consumption and cognitive impairment.

The authors wrote: "Given the high prevalence, worldwide rapid increase, and clinical significance of dementia... any association between the intake of green tea, a drink with little toxicity and no calorific value, and cognitive function could have considerable clinical and public health relevance."

... Green tea could help put a stop to the maddening itching and persistent pain caused by psoriasis

If the results of the latest findings from an animal study, conducted by US researchers from the Medical College of Georgia, are anything to go by then green tea could prove effective when applied topically to skin afflicted by inflammatory disorders such as psoriasis and dandruff (*Experimental Dermatology, 18 August 2007*).

At present, psoriasis – an irritating skin condition that causes raised red patches of skin to appear on the body – affects around 2 per cent of people in the UK. It strikes both sexes equally and can arise at any age, although it is more likely to appear between the ages of 11 and 45.

The unsightly appearance of these lesions can soon leave sufferers feeling isolated and depressed. To make matters worse, the lesions are often inflamed and itchy, sometimes to the point of preventing sleep or concentration on normal activities.

Lead researcher, Dr Stephen Hsu, an oral biologist at the Medical College of Georgia's School of Dentistry and Maxillofacial Pathology, explained that: "Psoriasis, an autoimmune disease, causes the skin to become thicker because the growth of skin cells is out of control. In psoriasis, immune cells, which usually protect against infection, instead trigger the release of cytokines, which causes inflammation and the overproduction of skin cells."

For the purpose of the study, Dr Hsu and his colleagues examined the influence of green tea extract on the molecular pathways of animals with inflammatory skin disease. The researchers discovered that green tea regulates the expression of a protein known as caspase-14, which controls the skin cells' life cycle.

Dr Hsu explained: "That marker guides cells by telling them when to differentiate, die off and form a skin barrier. In people with psoriasis, that process is interrupted and the skin cells don't die before more are created and the resulting lesions form."

Dr Shu hopes that his team's research with green tea will contribute to a treatment that has less side effects than current treatments for inflammatory skin conditions. As Dr Hsu points out: "The traditional treatment of ultraviolet light and medication, while it can control the lesions and be used long term, may cause squamous cell carcinoma – the second most common form of skin cancer," he said. "Some of the most effective anti-dandruff shampoos also have carcinogens in them. While the US Food and Drug Administration allows that in small amounts, the bottom line is that we don't know the long-term effects of using those products continuously."

... Simply drinking a cup of green tea each day could help prevent an allergy attack

Japanese researchers have discovered that drinking green tea has therapeutic benefits for allergy sufferers.

The researchers found that a compound present in green tea – epigallocatechin gallate (EGCG) – is able to block the formation of two compounds that can trigger an allergic reaction: histamine and immunoglobulin E (IgE). For example, these compounds have been found to be responsible for causing dust mite allergies and food intolerances in susceptible individuals.

By studying the human white blood cells that release histamine, called basophils, the researchers found that a methylated form of EGCG inhibits the IgE receptor, involved in an allergic response.

Methylated EGCG appears to provide a more powerful response than normal EGCG against allergies. The researchers believe this is why green tea provides such an effective anti-allergy effect, as it contains high amounts of methylated EGCG.

Dr Hirofumi Tachibana (Associate Professor of Chemistry at Kyushu University in Fukuoka, Japan), who led the study, stated: "Green tea appears to be a promising source for effective anti-allergenic agents. If you have allergies, you should consider drinking it."

... Latest research findings reveal anti-cancer benefit linked to green tea

There really does appear to be no end to green tea's long list of health benefits. Scientists have found that it's effective against many different types of cancers, including those affecting the prostate, stomach, pancreas, breast, lung and colon.

Now a new study has found another type of cancer that green tea can help fight – oesophageal cancer. The oesophagus is the muscular tube that propels food from your mouth to your stomach. In particular, the researchers found that green tea is able to inhibit oesophageal cancer associated with a condition called Barrett's oesophagus – chronic irritation of the oesophagus caused by heartburn and acid reflux.

Dr Howard Y Chang and colleagues who conducted the study at the Harvard Medical School and the Veterans Administration Boston Healthcare System in the US, recently presented their findings at the Digestive Disease Week convention, held in New Orleans.

They believe that the oesophagus may benefit from being exposed to high levels of polyphenols, such as epigallocatechin gallate

(EGCG), which are present in green tea. Polyphenols are natural chemicals that have antioxidant properties – this means they're able to fight harmful free radicals that can damage cells. EGCG in particular, is believed to block the production of an enzyme needed for cancer cells to grow. It is also thought to suppress the production of blood vessels that supply blood to cancer cells.

The scientists administered varying concentrations of EGCG to human Barrett's oesophagus-associated adenocarcinoma (cancerous) cells in the laboratory, and compared them to untreated cells. They found that cell growth was inhibited within 72 hours after exposure to EGCG. The team concluded that EGCG also induced cell death, which occurred as early as 24 hours after the treated cells were exposed to the compound.

Commenting on the results, Dr Chang said: "Research suggests that drinking green tea may be both a valuable chemopreventive therapy as well as a treatment for oesophageal adenocarcinoma. Our results suggest that extracts in green tea may help to lower the prevalence of oesophageal adenocarcinoma, one of the fastest growing cancers in Western countries."

Other types of beneficial teas

Ginger tea

According to Traditional Chinese Medicine ginger tea is an excellent way to prevent indigestion. It is also effective against nausea.

Peppermint tea

Follow the French tradition and end your meal not with coffee but a pot of peppermint tea – which has a strong calming action on your gut. Peppermint is a relatively new remedy – the plant only having been cultivated in the last 300 years. Since then, herbalists have used it as a remedy to relieve IBS symptoms like indigestion and nausea.

Dandelion tea

Because of the high vitamin A and C content in dandelion leaves, they help your body repair damaged tissue and help your liver clear toxins from the blood.

Nettle leaf tea

Nettle leaf extracts have been found to block a chemical called TNF (Tumour Necrosis Factor), which is responsible for destroying tissues within your joints (*FEBS Lett 1999 442(1) 89-94*). The extract of the leaf also influences chemicals, such as the enzyme cyclooxygenase, which is involved in the inflammatory process.

Fennel tea

Fennel herbal tea is a good choice if you suffer from gout, colic or intestinal gas. It also acts as a gentle diuretic.

Camomile tea

This is an excellent choice of beverage if you suffer from anxiety, insomnia, headaches or digestive problems. This is because camomile has a calming effect which works on your entire system.

The compound that a leading Harvard medical professor believes 'could potentially get rid of 4 out of the 5 most common diseases in the Western world'

An ingredient found in cocoa, tea and wine is currently causing a great deal of excitement among scientists for its potential to ward off a wide range of chronic diseases.

In fact, Harvard Medical School Professor of Medicine Norman Hollenberg believes that epicatechin is so important that it should be considered a vitamin (*Chemistry and Industry, 12 March 2007*).

Dr Hollenberg's conviction is based upon observations of the Kuna people of Panama, who drink up to 40 cups of cocoa per week. The risk of some of the most common Western diseases: stroke, heart failure, cancer and diabetes, is reduced to less than 10 per cent in this population. Additionally, no cases of dementia have been observed among their elderly population.

"If these observations predict the future, then we can say without blushing that they are among the most important observations in the history of medicine," Dr Hollenberg stated. "We all agree that penicillin and anaesthesia are enormously important. But epicatechin could potentially get rid of four of the five most common diseases in the Western world, how important does that make epicatechin?... I would say very important."

While many individuals might look forward to a guilt-free mug of hot chocolate, "no doubt some people would prefer to get their epicatechin in capsule form," Dr Hollenberg noted.

In response to Dr Hollenberg's comments, Daniel Fabricant, Vice President of Scientific Affairs at the Natural Products Association, said: "Vitamins are defined as being essential to the normal functioning, metabolism, regulation and growth of cells. At the moment, the science does not support epicatechin having an essential role." However, he added that "the link between high epicatechin consumption and a decreased risk of killer disease is so striking, it should be investigated further. It may be that these diseases are the result of epicatechin deficiency."

Alcohol can be a major obstacle in the battle to lose weight

While there are certain health benefits attached to drinking some alcoholic beverages, the best advice if you enjoy a drink is to do so in moderation. The reason for this is that alcohol upsets blood sugar levels, depletes nutrients, causes liver problems, aggravates the gut, lowers immunity and, if you're trying to lose weight it is not good news as it increases hunger and cravings for junk foods.

If you do like alcohol then opt for red wine. Many of you will probably be aware that some doctors actually encourage patients to drink a glass or two of red or white wine each day, because it is a potent source of antioxidants, known as flavonoids. There is good evidence to show moderate drinkers are healthier and live longer than tee-totallers because of these healthful properties.

There is also a beneficial antioxidant found in wine, resveratrol, which is present in grape skins (red grapes have higher concentrations than white, which is why red wine is a healthier option than white wine). Grapes produce resveratrol in response to infestation with a fungus (grey mould) called *Botrytis cinerea*. When the grape skins are macerated (crushed) during the wine making process, the concentration of resveratrol increases tenfold.

Its claim to fame is connected with the 'French Paradox', namely the low numbers of patients with heart disease in France, despite their consumption of a high fat diet (*Biochem Pharmacol 1998; 55: 811-6*). The theory is that the French have a low risk of heart disease because they drink red wine with every meal, and this acts as the antidote against the risks of a high fat diet (*Eur J Endocrinol 1998; 138: 619-20*).

Lowers LDL cholesterol and prevents abnormal clotting

There are dozens of scientific studies which suggest that drinking a moderate amount of red wine may reduce the risk of coronary heart disease that can lead to a heart attack. Resveratrol is an effective antioxidant which protects the muscles of the heart against toxic poisons created during normal metabolism.

Resveratrol works by preventing the damage caused by low-density lipoprotein or LDL (the 'bad' cholesterol). It also prevents any abnormal clotting of the blood, and so it reduces the risk of a blockage in the arteries of the heart (*Eur J Cardiovasc Prev Rehabil 2005; 12(6): 596-600*).

May be useful in the fight against breast, bowel and liver cancers

Recent research shows that resveratrol may be a useful plant chemical to use against several types of cancer. Resveratrol is thought to work in a variety of ways to reduce the likelihood of cancer.

For example, it can help block the supply of blood to the cancerous growth, thereby causing any cancer to wither and die. It also, for some unknown reason, attacks and destroys cancerous cells while at the same time allowing normal healthy cells to remain unharmed.

In a study published by researchers from the Faculty of Health Sciences, University Hospital, Linköping in Sweden, the scientists observed a significantly lower breast cancer growth in cells treated with resveratrol. The scientists concluded that their study "supports the potential use of resveratrol as a chemotherapeutic agent in breast cancer" (*Cancer Lett 2006; 231(1):113-22*).

A new study shows that substances found in beer, wine and tea could prevent the spread of breast cancer

The results of a study on breast cancer were announced by Portuguese scientists at the Experimental Biology 2004 meeting held in Washington in the US. What makes their research findings so extraordinary is that they contradict earlier study results showing that alcohol increases the risk of the disease.

The latest study conducted at the Universidade do Porto in Portugal, revealed how certain compounds called phenolic phytochemicals – found in wine, beer (and tea) – were able to help stop the growth of human breast cancer cells in the laboratory.

In particular the scientists investigated three phenolic compounds: epigallocatechin gallate (EGCG), which is found in tea (as mentioned on page 224); xanthohumol (XN) found in beer; and resveratrol (RES) found in red wine.

All three compounds were found to significantly slow down the spread of breast cancer cells. This effect was most pronounced in the case of XN found in beer, which worked more quickly than the other two compounds tested and at a lower concentration. EGCG found in tea exhibited the least potent effect against breast cancer, although it was also found to be the least toxic compound – which according to the researchers means it can be given in higher doses.

The researchers were quick to point out that their findings should not encourage women to increase their alcohol consumption in an attempt to prevent breast cancer until further studies are conducted which confirm these results.

Other scientists recently reported beneficial results of resveratrol in bowel cancer. They found that resveratrol works in different stages of bowel cancer and blocks several steps in the development of that cancer (*Sengottuvelan M, et. al. Carcinogenesis, published online 7 December 2005*).

Working along the same principles, French researchers from the University Victor Segalen in Bordeaux reported that resveratrol is also active against liver cancer in humans (*Int J Biochem Cell Biol 2006; 38(4): 629-37*). They believe that resveratrol blocks the chemical signals between cancerous cells. This confuses their growth patterns and does not allow them to multiply.

Finally, certain scientists believe that resveratrol works by making cancer cells more sensitive to conventional chemotherapy drugs (*Antioxid Redox Signal 2005; 7(11-12): 1630-47*).

Could resveratrol have possible anti-ageing properties?

People keen in learning about anti-ageing medicine know that calorie restriction is an effective treatment against ageing. Calorie restriction simply means to consume around 30 per cent less calories than what is considered a 'normal' amount. This activates certain genes, which manufacture natural chemicals that fight the ageing process within your cells.

The problem is that not many people want to spend a lifetime on a constant and strict diet just to gain a few extra years of life. But cutting-edge research shows that the same genes activated by calorie restriction can also be activated by using certain specific chemicals called Calorie Restriction Mimetics (i.e. compounds that give you the same benefits of a calorie restriction diet, but without the need to actually go on a diet). Calorie restriction treatment works by activating the SIR-2 gene, a crucial life-extending gene.

One of these compounds is resveratrol. It turns out that resveratrol activates the SIR-2 gene (*Dev Cell 2005; 9(5): 605-15*). Research shows that, in yeast, resveratrol stimulates the SIR-2 gene and strengthens the DNA which extends lifespan by 70 per cent (*Curr Opin Chem Biol 2005; 9(5): 431-40*).

There are several other scientific studies that support the use of resveratrol as an alternative to a lifelong diet in order to increase lifespan. Unfortunately, the majority of these studies have been performed on animals in the laboratory, but scientists believe that the same results must hold true for humans too. It will be another few years before research on humans will confirm this beyond doubt.

But if it turns out to be true it would mean that compounds like resveratrol are not only affective against heart disease and cancer, but also against the ageing process itself, helping us to live longer.

What to take for best results

So how much resveratrol do you need to receive these protective benefits? A glass of red wine provides about 640 micrograms but resveratrol supplements are available too if you prefer not to get your RDA from an alcoholic source. The recommended dose is 200-600 micrograms daily.

A final word of advice

By regularly eating a wide selection of the super foods outlined in *Super Foods for a Super Healthy You*, you should start to look and feel better in no time. Plus, by eating such highly nutritious foods you'll be arming your body with what it needs to help prevent and treat all kinds of ailments – from Alzheimer's to arthritis.

After reading *Super Foods for a Super Healthy You* you'll have all the tools you need to help you fine-tune your diet to get the very most from the foods you already consume, while introducing other, powerful, therapeutic foods to help you achieve 'optimum' health.

Best of all, the majority of these 'super foods' aren't difficult to source or expensive... in fact, most are common vegetables, fruits, seeds and herbs that you'll find lining supermarket shelves up and down the country.

Try adding different 'super foods' to your shopping list each time you pop to the supermarket and then incorporate them into the delicious and nutritious recipes listed. A helpful reference guide listing different dishes to suit your specific needs is provided on page 243 – you'll find easy-to-prepare recipes for when you're in a rush, those that are suitable for vegetarians, recipes to suit the different seasons and those that are perfect for entertaining guests. But don't feel limited to these alone – experiment with different 'super food' combinations.

Variety really is the key here to making the right food choices that are fundamental to helping you achieve a long and healthy life.

Bon appetite!

FURTHER READING:

S uperFoods. Fourteen Foods That Will Change Your Life by Steven Pratt, MD and Kathy Matthews (Bantam Books, ISBN: 0553817639). Doctor Steven Pratt divulges the top 14 nutrient-dense foods he believes can slow down or stop the incremental changes in your body that lead to diseases like diabetes and Alzheimer's when eaten on a regular basis.

Dr Gillian McKeith's Living Food for Health: 12 Natural Superfoods to Transform Your Health by Dr Gillian McKeith (Piatkus, ISBN: 074992540X). International nutritionist Dr Gillian McKeith gives advice on the 12 foods she believes can transform your health and well-being, from boosting your energy levels to improving your digestion.

Miracle Foods: 25 Super-Nutritious Foods For Great Health by Anna Selby (Hamlyn, ISBN: 0600610829). Essential information on 25 key miracle foods, plus how to choose, store and use them.

Superfoods, Superfast by Michael Van Straten (Dorling Kindersley Publishers Ltd, ISBN-10: 405315598). This book helps you to discover how easy it is to prepare good food fast with 200 sumptuous recipes featuring over 90 nutridense superfoods packed with antioxidants, nutrients and vitamins.

Brain Food: The Essential Guide to Boosting Your Brain Power by Lorraine Perretta (Pyramid Paperbacks, ISBN-10: 0600610888). Identify the key IQ-boosting foods and discover how to fuel your brain and eat your way to exam success.

Power Food: For Energy and Strength by Janette Marshall (Pyramid Paperbacks, ISBN-10: 060061087X). This is a guide to how our bodies use the food we eat, which have the most nutritional value, and how and when we should be eating them. There are over 50 well-balanced recipes designed to help keep your energy levels up.

HELPFUL ORGANISATIONS:

Complementary Practitioners

The Guild of Complementary Practitioners (GCP)
Liddell House
Liddell Close
Finchamstead
Berkshire
RG40 4NS

Tel: 0118 973 5757
Website: www.gcpnet.com

Nutrition

The British Association of Nutritional Therapists
27 Old Gloucester Street
London
WC1N 3XX

You can obtain a list of registered nutritional therapists in your area by sending £2 to the above address

Supplements

The Nutri Centre
7 Park Crescent
London
W1B 1PF

Tel: 020 7436 5122

Your helpful recipe guide at a glance

The following guide is designed to help you select the recipes outlined in *Super Foods for a Super Healthy You* that best suit your needs at any given time, to save you from having to trawl back through the book trying to locate them.

Categorized into sections they'll help you decide which recipes are quick to prepare if you don't have much time on your hands... ensuring that you get fast food without compromising your health in the process.

You'll also find a list of warming dishes that are perfect for the cold winter months, and those menu ideas which are better suited to a hot summer's day... although obviously, this is by no means set in stone so feel free to alternate!

There's a list of dishes suitable for vegetarians, plus if you're entertaining or cooking for a special occasion, there's also a category devoted to delicious meals and desserts to wow your guests.

Tasty meals and drinks you can rustle up in 15 minutes or less

Refreshing açaí and mango smoothie – page 13
Pork chops with apple sauce – page 15
Spicy avocado dip to wake up your taste buds – page 19
Festive cranberry sauce – the perfect accompaniment to turkey – page 35
Simple-to-prepare pineapple salsa – page 38
The dark purple smoothie loaded with antioxidants – page 45
Berry bliss smoothie – page 47
Spicy chicken and broccoli dish – page 67
Steamed garlic and lemon grass sea bass – page 72
Spinach, avocado and beetroot salad – page 85

Kick-start your day with a refreshing fruit and oat smoothie – page 100
Tuna and butter bean salad – page 112
Mushroom and miso soup – page 113
Quick and delicious banana and cinnamon smoothie – page 123
Fresh fennel and walnut salad – page 126
Prawn and veggie ginger stir fry – page 128
Instant energy ginger juice – page 129
Black olives with oregano – page 133
Rosemary chicken with a kick – page 137
Broccoli and walnut salad with apple vinaigrette sauce – page 146
Sautéed sea bass with virgin coconut oil and garlic – page 156
Salad niçoise – page 167
Chicken caesar salad (please note, this recipe is quick to prepare if
you've pre-cooked the chicken in advance) – page 171
Pork and spinach sesame seed stir-fry – page 172
Grilled salmon fillets with a herb yoghurt – page 178
Pepper, lentil and goat's cheese surprise – page 179
Asparagus and sautéed mushroom-filled omelette – page 182

Winter warmers – The perfect comfort foods

Pork chops with apple sauce – page 15
Banana and raisin bread – page 21
Mouthwatering blueberry muffins – page 26
Festive cranberry sauce – the perfect accompaniment to turkey – page 35
Orange and lemon roasted chicken – page 36
Ratatouille – A traditional, tasty way to benefit from tomatoes – page 49
Spicy chicken and broccoli dish – page 67
Mixed oriental mushroom risotto – page 74
Vegetarian shepherd's pie with sweet potato – page 80
Hearty pumpkin, pepper and coriander soup – page 83
Quinoa and tofu loaf – page 98
Comforting lentil and tomato soup – page 111
Hearty split pea soup – page 111
Mushroom and miso soup – page 113

Chickpea casserole with spinach – page 114
Cod in tomato and basil sauce – page 119
Quick and delicious banana and cinnamon smoothie – page 123
Rosemary chicken with a kick – page 137
Spicy pumpkin curry with turmeric – page 141
Chunky nut and vegetable roast – page 147
This spicy mackerel dish provides a tasty way to top up your levels of omega-3 – page 162
Warming turkey chilli – page 170
Grilled salmon with a herb yoghurt sauce – page 178
Eggs Florentine and haddock – page 183
Roasted veg with manuka honey and feta cheese – page 189

When the temperature rises try these delicious summertime dishes

Refreshing açaí and mango smoothie – page 13
Spicy avocado dip to wake up your taste buds – page 19
Cherry sorbet – for the occasional tasty treat – page 30
Simple-to-prepare pineapple salsa – page 38
The dark purple smoothie loaded with antioxidants – page 45
Berry bliss smoothie – page 47
Delicious vegetarian sushi rolls – page 53
Beetroot soup – a delicious way to cleanse your system – page 65
Steamed garlic and lemon grass sea bass – page 72
Go continental with a delicious French onion tart – page 77
Spinach, avocado and beetroot salad – page 85
Watercress and goat's cheese salad – page 88
Savoury brown rice nutty salad – page 98
Spiced prawn, avocado and bulgar wheat salad with salmon pancake rolls – page 99
Kick-start your day with a refreshing fruit and oat smoothie – page 100
Tuna and butter bean salad – page 112
Fresh fennel and walnut salad – page 126
Prawn and veggie ginger stir-fry – page 128

Instant energy ginger juice – page 129
Black olives with oregano – page 133
Broccoli and walnut salad with apple vinaigrette sauce – page 146
Sautéed sea bass with virgin coconut oil and garlic – page 156
Roasted vegetables in extra virgin olive oil with couscous – page 157
Salmon with a tangy, mango salsa twist – page 164
Grilled oysters in lemon butter – page 165
Monkfish and veggie mix – page 166
Salad niçoise – page 167
Chicken caesar salad – page 171
Pork and spinach sesame seed stir-fry – page 172
Pepper, lentil and goat's cheese surprise – page 179
Asparagus and sautéed mushroom-filled omelette – page 182

Vegetarian super food options

Refreshing açaí and mango smoothie – page 13
Spicy avocado dip to wake up your taste buds – page 19
Banana and raisin bread – page 21
Mouthwatering blueberry muffins – page 26
Cherry sorbet – for the occasional tasty treat – page 30
Festive cranberry sauce – the perfect accompaniment to turkey – page 35
Simple-to-prepare pineapple salsa – page 38
The dark purple smoothie loaded with antioxidants – page 45
Berry bliss smoothie – page 47
Ratatouille – A traditional, tasty way to benefit from tomatoes – page 49
Delicious vegetarian sushi rolls – page 53
Beetroot soup – A delicious way to cleanse your system – page 65
Mixed oriental mushroom risotto – page 74
Go continental with a delicious French onion tart – page 77
Vegetarian shepherd's pie with sweet potato – page 80
Hearty pumpkin, pepper and coriander soup – page 83
Spinach, avocado and beetroot salad – page 85
Watercress and goat's cheese salad – page 88
Savoury brown rice nutty salad – page 98

Quinoa and tofu loaf – page 98
Kick-start your day with a refreshing fruit and oat smoothie – page 100
Comforting lentil and tomato soup – page 111
Hearty split pea soup (opt for the vegetable stock) – page 111
Chickpea casserole with spinach – page 114
Quick and delicious banana and cinnamon smoothie – page 123
Fresh fennel and walnut salad – page 126
Instant energy ginger juice – page 129
Black olives with oregano – page 133
Spicy pumpkin curry with turmeric – page 141
Broccoli and walnut salad with apple vinaigrette sauce – page 146
Chunky nut & vegetable roast – page 147
Roasted vegetables in extra virgin olive oil with couscous – page 157
Pepper, lentil and goat's cheese surprise – page 179
Asparagus and sautéed mushroom filled omelette – page 182
Roasted veg with manuka honey and feta cheese – page 189
Indulgent chocolate and walnut mousse – page 194

Meals for special occasions and entertaining

Starters and side dishes

Spicy avocado dip to wake up your taste buds – page 19
Black olives with oregano – page 133
Cherry sorbet – for the occasional tasty treat (suitable both as a starter
and a dessert) – page 30
Beetroot soup – a delicious way to cleanse your system – page 65
Hearty pumpkin, pepper and coriander soup – page 83
Comforting lentil and tomato soup – page 111
Hearty split pea soup – page 111
Mushroom and miso soup – page 113
Spinach, avocado and beetroot salad – page 85
Watercress and goat's cheese salad – page 88
Fresh fennel and walnut salad – page 126
Salad niçoise – page 167

Chicken caesar salad – page 171
Pepper, lentil and goat's cheese surprise – page 179
Roasted veg with manuka honey and feta cheese – page 189
Grilled oysters in lemon butter – page 165

Main

Festive cranberry sauce – the perfect accompaniment to turkey – page 35
Orange and lemon roasted chicken – page 36
Rosemary chicken with a kick – page 137
Spicy pumpkin curry with turmeric – page 141
Roasted vegetables in extra virgin olive oil with couscous – page 157
Chunky nut and vegetable roast – page 147
Simple-to-prepare pineapple salsa (perfect fish accompaniment) – page 38
Steamed garlic and lemon grass sea bass – page 72
Sautéed sea bass with virgin coconut oil and garlic – page 156
Monkfish and veggie mix – page 166
Salmon with a tangy, mango salsa twist – page 164
Grilled salmon fillets with a herb yoghurt sauce – page 178
Spiced prawn, avocado and bulgar wheat salad with salmon pancake rolls – page 99

Dessert

Cherry sorbet – for the occasional tasty treat (suitable both as a starter and a dessert) – page 30
Indulgent chocolate and walnut mousse – page 194

INDEX

A

Açaí 10, 11, 12, 13
Ageing 10,16, 23, 53, 60, 78, 79, 106, 136, 226, 237, 238
Age-related macular degeneration (ARMD) 85, 161, 162
Alcohol..............3, 51, 94, 174, 199, 212, 221, 222, 234, 236, 238
Allergies..........73, 91, 146, 174, 176, 197, 198, 199 212, 229, 230
Aluminium...205, 206, 207
Alzheimer's 2, 61, 125, 160, 181, 205, 206, 207,
....224, 225, 226, 227, 239, 240
Antioxidants.......................4, 7, 8, 10, 17, 23, 24, 28, 32, 42, 45,
....53, 55, 60, 78, 82, 86, 94, 108, 124,
....130, 134, 143, 145, 218, 234, 240
Apples................6, 8, 14, 15, 29, 42, 43, 52, 56, 96, 120, 146, 191
Arthritis 4, 27, 84, 127, 130, 140, 212, 239
Ashitaba 58, 59, 60, 61
Asthma 14, 117, 130, 134, 174, 197, 212
Avocados..15, 18, 19, 96, 99, 149, 150

B

Bananas..9, 15, 20, 21, 22, 56, 78, 96, 216
Basil 117, 118, 119
Beans..........................56, 62, 68, 77, 94, 103, 104, 105, 112, 177
Beer 236
Beta-carotene 17, 18, 36, 59, 79, 81, 86, 87, 117
Bioflavoniods 7, 84
Bladder cancer 14
Blood pressure............................4, 19, 20, 27, 36, 39, 59, 60, 62,
....64, 65, 69, 84, 104, 146, 157,
....174, 175, 182, 192, 193, 212
Blood sugar levels....................1, 14, 61, 73, 81, 82, 93, 104, 106,
....120, 121, 122, 192, 217, 221, 234
Blueberries...............7, 11, 12, 22, 23, 24, 25, 26, 39, 47, 220, 221

Boron..14
Bowel cancer..............................2, 127, 128, 146, 176, 236, 237
Brazil nuts...145, 147, 177
Breast cancer........................85, 104, 105, 135, 146, 152, 235, 236
Broccoli.........................8, 15, 23, 55, 66, 67, 68, 79, 146, 177
Buckwheat...97

C

Calcium.....................20, 34, 36, 38, 51, 59, 63, 72, 76, 81, 84, 85,
.................................86, 96, 97, 108, 118, 173, 176, 177, 217, 222
Camomile tea...232
Cancer........................2, 3, 4, 5, 7, 8, 9, 10, 11, 12, 14, 17, 18, 19,
...........22, 23, 24, 35, 36, 39, 40, 41, 43, 46, 47, 48, 49, 53, 55, 60,
...........63, 66, 67, 70, 73, 74, 76, 78, 79, 81, 84, 85, 86, 87, 88, 93,
............95, 104, 105, 127, 128, 130, 133, 134, 135, 146, 150, 152,
............153, 169, 174, 176, 177, 202, 203, 216, 218, 223, 224, 229,
.................................230, 231, 233, 235, 236, 237, 238
Candida..176
Cataracts..81, 85
Celery...4, 9, 15, 58, 60, 62, 68
Cheese..................................88, 176, 177, 179, 189
Cherries...................................15, 27, 28, 29, 30
Chicken.................................36, 67, 137, 171
Chickpeas...56, 114
Chocolate.........................6, 192, 193, 194, 212
Cholesterol........................9, 11, 12, 13, 14, 18, 27, 28, 32, 36, 59,
.................................60, 63, 70, 71, 76, 81, 92, 93, 94, 97, 104,
.................................109, 117, 143, 144, 145, 149, 150, 153, 181,
.................................192, 194, 208, 212, 235
Cinnamon.........................1, 120, 121, 122, 123, 130
Coconut oil...........................153, 154, 155, 156
Cod...119
Coffee............................199, 212, 217, 218, 219, 220,
.................................221, 222, 223, 225, 227
Colds...................................51, 127, 138, 176, 187

Colon cancer...............................14, 76, 84, 93, 152, 153, 177, 218
Constipation..........................21, 84, 104, 106, 107, 139, 212
Cooking utensils 205
Copper 59, 73, 81, 108
Coughs.......................................123, 130, 187
Cranberries 8, 9, 23, 31, 32, 33, 34, 35
Cystitis...22, 23

D

Dairy 153, 173, 174, 175, 176, 177, 198
Dandelion tea 232
Dark chocolate.................................192, 193, 194
Diabetes 1, 2, 14, 27, 28, 59, 61, 76, 78, 82,
..........................92, 94, 95, 96, 106, 120, 121, 122, 149, 191,
....192, 212, 217, 218, 233, 240
Diarrhoea.....................21, 51, 91, 124, 125, 130, 132, 139,
....141, 154, 174, 176, 197, 199
Drinks...212, 216, 222, 243

E

Eggs 59, 62, 133, 181, 182, 183, 199, 216
Elimination diet...198, 199
Ellagitannins 39, 40, 42, 44, 45, 46, 47, 220
Exercise...2, 4, 28, 29, 30, 174, 175

F

Fats 3, 58, 106, 143, 149, 150, 152,
....153, 154, 155, 159, 169, 191, 192
Fennel.....................................9, 61, 123, 124, 125, 126
Fennel tea 232
Fibre...............................11, 12, 14, 15, 18, 20, 21, 36, 43, 55, 56,
...............................62, 63, 72, 78, 79, 81, 84, 85, 91, 92, 93,
.............................94, 95, 96, 97, 103, 104, 107, 110, 146
Fish 1, 2, 59, 107, 108, 123, 133, 149, 150,
.......................151, 152, 159, 160, 161, 162, 166, 177, 199, 208

Flavonoids 8, 9, 14, 33, 34, 39, 63, 85, 118, 124,
..............................130, 134, 192, 193, 194, 219, 234
Flaxseed 103, 104, 107, 152
Flu 51, 154
Fluoride 205, 206, 207, 215, 216, 217
Folate 8, 18, 85, 110, 144
Folic acid 36, 59, 63, 84, 85, 86, 181
Food allergy 197, 198, 199
Food intolerance.........................140, 197, 198, 229
Food poisoning 51, 125, 131, 133
Fruit 2, 4, 6, 7, 9, 10, 11
Fungal infections..69, 130

G

Garlic..............................9, 23, 59, 68, 69, 70, 71, 72, 156
Ginger 127, 128, 129, 138
Ginger tea 231
Goat's cheese 88, 176, 179
Gout 27, 232
Grains..............................4, 12, 91, 92, 94, 106, 150
Green tea.........39, 51, 61, 223, 225, 226, 227, 228, 229, 230, 231

H

Haddock 151, 183
Heart disease 2, 3, 5, 8, 9, 10, 12, 22, 23, 24, 32,
..............................52, 55, 70, 71, 76, 78, 79, 81, 84, 85, 94, 103,
..............................104, 121, 130, 134, 143, 144, 146, 149, 159,
..............................160, 169, 174, 181, 192, 193, 212, 234, 235, 238
Hemp seed oil 105, 106, 149, 151
Herbs..............................61, 117, 123, 130, 132, 239
Honey..............................6, 51, 185, 186, 187, 188, 189, 191

I

Immunity 31, 59, 66, 110, 143, 223, 234
Iron 18, 51, 59, 63, 72, 78, 81, 84, 86, 96,
...................................97, 108, 110, 118, 146, 169, 182
Irritable bowel syndrome (IBS)..........................91, 96, 138, 198

J

K

L

Lentils 56, 110, 111, 179
Libido 124
Lung cancer...7, 14, 127
Lutein 8, 18, 81, 84, 85, 87

M

Mackerel 151, 160, 162
Magnesium 36, 59, 62, 63, 81, 85, 94, 95, 108,
....110, 117, 146, 173, 182, 201, 217
Manganese 20, 59, 63, 81
Manuka honey 185, 186, 188, 189
Meat..................................2, 52, 59, 62, 133, 169, 170, 201, 216
Mediterranean diet..144, 150
Memory................................25, 85, 124, 160, 223, 225, 226, 227
Menopause..104, 124, 220
Metabolic syndrome...27, 28
Microwaves 207, 208, 209
Migraines 182, 197, 198
Milk.............................21, 86, 103, 105, 124, 133, 154, 173,
....174, 175, 176, 177, 197, 199, 216
Miso...50, 105, 113
Monkfish 166
MRSA...185, 188
Mushrooms..............................9, 72, 73, 74, 75, 96, 113, 182

N

Nettle leaf tea..232
Nuts 1, 4, 62, 94, 98, 143, 144, 146, 149, 150, 151, 160, 199

O

Oats 91, 94, 96
Oesophageal cancer...230
Olive oil..........................10, 11, 144, 145, 149, 150, 151, 152, 157
Omega-3 fatty acids...........................97, 104, 105, 106, 107, 108,
....145, 151, 159, 160, 161, 162
Omega-6 fatty acids 11, 105, 106, 151
Onions...8, 9, 15, 68, 69, 75, 76, 77
Oranges 7, 35, 36, 86, 96
Oregano 130, 131, 132, 133
Organic...........................4, 10, 15, 169, 175, 201, 202, 203
Osteoarthritis 2, 117, 152
Osteoporosis 5, 14, 75, 76, 84, 85, 173, 216
Oysters..162, 165

P

Pancreatitis...221, 222
Pasta 56, 91, 92, 117
Peanuts..11, 144
Pectin 14, 21, 36
Peppermint tea..231
Phosphorus 81, 108
Phytonutrients 14, 18, 19
Pineapple.....................................7, 15, 37, 38, 216
Pomegranates 8, 39, 40, 42, 43, 44, 217, 218, 220
Pork..15, 153, 169, 172
Potassium 9, 18, 20, 21, 36, 51, 59, 62, 63, 78,
....81, 108, 110, 118, 137, 182
Potatoes...............7, 11, 15, 56, 68, 72, 78, 79, 96
Prawns 99, 128
Prostate cancer 9, 14, 41, 48, 49, 73, 74, 146

Protein 21, 38, 49, 56, 72, 81, 85, 93, 94, 97,
.................................103, 104, 107, 109, 110, 136, 143, 146, 169,
.................................175, 177, 181, 199, 208, 225, 226, 229
Psoriasis..156, 228, 229
Pulses 56, 103, 110, 213
Pumpkin.............................81, 82, 83, 96, 110, 141, 174

Q
Quercetin.............................14, 23, 33, 34, 76, 108, 124
Quinoa...97, 98

R
Raspberries 15, 40, 46, 47, 220, 221
Resveratrol..............................234, 235, 236, 237, 238
Rheumatoid arthritis 27, 117, 119, 152, 197
Rice 50, 53, 94, 96, 97, 98, 175
Rosemary...............................133, 134, 135, 136, 137

S
Salba seeds 106, 109
Salmon 99, 107, 151, 160, 164, 177, 178
Salt (sodium) 3, 20, 27, 56, 137, 174, 176, 212
Seabass 72, 156
Selenium 110, 146, 169, 201
Sesame seeds..68, 110, 172
Soy/Soya...........................103, 104, 105, 174, 175, 199
Spices 117, 120, 127, 128
Spinach..........7, 8, 15, 23, 25, 59, 61, 63, 68, 84, 85, 86, 114, 172
Split peas..111
Stomach ulcers 21, 60, 66, 154
Stroke 55, 62, 78, 117, 121, 143, 149, 181,
.................................191, 192, 202, 212, 233
Sugar............................2, 3, 5, 6, 44, 52, 56, 95, 96, 149,
.................................174, 185, 191, 192, 199, 212, 220
Super bugs 185

Sweet potatoes 7, 11, 68, 79, 80, 96

T

Tannins 23, 39, 44
Tea 23, 39, 58, 61, 127, 132, 185, 193, 212, 216, 222,
..................223, 224, 225, 226, 227, 228, 229, 230, 231, 232, 236
Teeth 33, 34, 36, 216
Thiamin...36
Tomatoes 8, 17, 48, 49, 50, 111, 119
Tofu 50, 98, 105, 213
Tuna...112, 159, 160
Turkey..35, 169, 170
Turmeric...138, 139, 140, 141

U

Urinary tract infections 9, 31, 131

V

Vegetables 2, 4, 6, 7, 8, 9, 10, 11, 15, 16, 17, 19, 23,
....25, 50, 53, 55, 56, 57, 58, 62, 64, 68, 72,
....84, 88, 92, 94, 96, 112, 156, 157, 160,
...............................174, 177, 193, 199, 202, 203, 213, 216, 239
Vitamin A 17, 79, 86, 117, 232
Vitamin B...20, 36, 59, 63, 207
Vitamin C................................4, 7, 17, 18, 20, 23, 35, 38, 59, 62,
....72, 78, 79, 81, 84, 86, 118, 185
Vitamin D 181
Vitamin E...17, 18, 42, 57, 58, 79, 134, 146

W

Walnuts 6, 21, 126, 144, 145, 146, 194
Water 64, 205, 206, 211, 212, 213, 214, 215, 216
Watercress...7, 8, 86, 87, 88
Watermelon 8, 17
Weight loss 4, 15, 36, 91, 92, 153, 155, 224

Wine 10, 11, 12, 39, 150, 193, 219, 232, 234, 235, 236, 238
Wounds...78, 185, 186, 188

X

Y

Yoghurt...105, 109, 176, 177, 178

Z

Zinc 59, 72, 81, 96, 108, 110, 162, 169, 182, 201